STUDYING HEALTH INEQUALITIES
An applied approach

Jonathan Wistow
with
Tim Blackman, David Byrne and Gerald Wistow

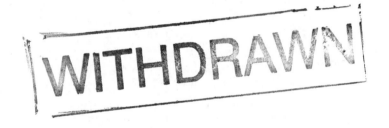

First published in Great Britain in 2015 by

Policy Press
University of Bristol
1-9 Old Park Hill
Bristol
BS2 8BB
UK
t: +44 (0)117 954 5940
pp-info@bristol.ac.uk
www.policypress.co.uk

North America office:
Policy Press
c/o The University of Chicago Press
1427 East 60th Street
Chicago, IL 60637, USA
t: +1 773 702 7700
f: +1 773-702-9756
sales@press.uchicago.edu
www.press.uchicago.edu

© Policy Press 2015
Reprinted 2015

British Library Cataloguing in Publication Data
A catalogue record for this book is available from the British Library

Library of Congress Cataloging-in-Publication Data
A catalog record for this book has been requested

ISBN 978 1 44730 528 6 hardcover
ISBN 978 1 44730 527 9 paperback

The right of Jonathan Wistow, Tim Blackman, David Byrne and Gerald Wistow to
be identified as authors of this work has been asserted by them in accordance with the
Copyright, Designs and Patents Act 1988.

Cover design by Soapbox
Front cover image: iStock
Printed and bound in Great Britain by www.4edge.co.uk
Policy Press uses environmentally responsible print partners

Contents

List of tables and figures

Tables

Figures

About the authors

Chris Bentley, FRCP FFPH. As a London qualified doctor, Chris migrated into population health via practice in East Africa (with Save the Children Fund and UNICEF), London, Sussex and Sheffield/South Yorkshire, where he was director of public health. He headed up the Health Inequalities National Support Team, which worked with the 70 most deprived areas of England with the poorest health (Spearhead areas), and based on this work provided ongoing policy advice to the Department of Health on population health issues. He now works independently, with contracts at local, regional and national level, and with WHO in Europe. He is a non-executive director of Derbyshire Community Healthcare NHS Trust, and is a visiting professor at Sheffield Hallam University.

Tim Blackman is vice-chancellor of Middlesex University London. He has held chairs in sociology and social policy at The Open University and Durham, Teesside and Oxford Brookes universities, and worked for several years as a government adviser on tackling health inequalities. He began his academic career at the University of Ulster where he undertook research on housing and health, which became a long-standing academic and policy interest.

David Byrne is professor of sociology and social policy in the School of Applied Social Sciences at Durham University. He has worked as an academic and in community development, and has been an inner-city municipal councillor. His interests are in the transition from industrial to post-industrial society and in the methodological programme of the social sciences, as this can be applied to understanding social issues and helping social action. He has published widely on these subjects.

Peter Counsell, MA MA MBA. Peter's career as a general manager spanned the voluntary and statutory sectors in social work, healthcare and public health at local, regional and national levels. He was the cancer lead in the HINST, leading the collaborative work with National Cancer Action Team

Gerald Wistow has been visiting professor in social policy at the London School of Economics and Political Science since 2004. He has previously been co-director of the Centre for Social Policy Research at Loughborough University, professor of health and social care management and director of the Nuffield Institute for Health at the University of Leeds, and visiting professor at the University of Durham. External roles have included appointments as a scientific adviser to the Department of Health, chair of a primary care trust and specialist adviser to the House of Commons Health Committee. He has published extensively on a wide range of health and social care issues

Jonathan Wistow is a lecturer in applied social sciences at Durham University. He has worked as a research fellow and research associate at Durham University on projects focusing on health inequalities, on health and social care systems and on climate change resilience and adaptation. Previously he worked in local government as a scrutiny support officer.

Preface

This book has its origins in a National Institute for Health Research Service Delivery and Organisation-funded research project ('Towards a new understanding of how local action can effectively address health inequalities') that was conducted between 2007 and 2009.[1] The project focused on health inequality targets to be met by 2010 for 70 Spearhead local authority areas in England with the worst health and deprivation. The project sought to explore what combinations of practice and context are associated with most progress towards the target. Further details about the project (including the final report) can be found at: www.nets.nihr.ac.uk/projects/hsdr/081716203.

The project was designed by Tim Blackman (principal investigator) and David Byrne (co-investigator), building on their expertise in complexity theory, health policy analysis and qualitative comparative analysis. Jonathan Wistow joined the project as research fellow. This book has been heavily influenced by the ontological and epistemological approach developed through the project. Although some time has elapsed since the original research took place, our analysis of more recent developments in policy, alongside broader methodological considerations, ensures the relevance of the book to contemporary debates.

Jonathan Wistow prepared the outline for the book. Full first draft chapters were written by individual authors. Jonathan Wistow was responsible for the first drafts of Chapters One, Two, Six, Eight and Nine; Tim Blackman for Chapter Three; David Byrne for Chapter Four; Gerald Wistow for Chapter Five; and Chris Bentley and Peter Counsell for Chapter Seven. Jonathan Wistow carried out the final edit of the book and would like to thank Gerald Wistow for his detailed comments on many of the chapters. As a result of the joint authorship of this book there is inevitably some variation in the style of writing across different chapters. However, there is much common ground between the authors in how we view and conceptualise health inequalities. The differences in perspective provide complementary rather than competing lenses through which to view this complex and wicked problem.

ONE

Introduction

Health outcomes in England are profoundly unequal. They exist between social groups and within and between geographical areas. Moreover, they are increasingly recognised to be indicative of wider and deeper social problems. According to Wilkinson and Pickett:

> It has been known for some years that poor health and violence are more common in more unequal societies. However, in the course of our research we became aware that almost all problems which are more common at the bottom of the social ladder are more common in more unequal societies. It is not just ill–health and violence, but also ... a host of other social problems. Almost all of them contribute to the widespread concern that modern societies are, despite their affluence, social failures. (2010: 18)

From this perspective, health inequalities can be viewed as both a cause and a consequence of the distribution of resources in different societies. Consequently, evidence about them can be seen to provide an interesting and important insight into the dynamics of contemporary societies. Health inequalities reflect (among other things) the way that we live our lives, the way that services are organised, the quality of service delivery, the history of places, the distribution of wealth, where people want to live, where people actually live and the opportunities and options people have throughout their different life stages. Since they both reflect and help to shape differences in our life chances, how does public policy seek to mitigate their impact and how successfully has it done so? These are two of the basic issues which this book is designed to address.

Having briefly set out our starting point, the remainder of this introductory chapter will contain a short discussion about different conceptions of health inequalities. It moves on to identify and outline potential causes of health inequalities, discussing the wider determinants of health and health inequalities and indicators of these. It also introduces issues about the nature and organisation of the public health function in England, where much of the policy debate about

1

health inequalities has been situated in recent years, and concludes by outlining the structure of the remaining chapters.

What are health inequalities?

Health inequalities have become a more central concern of public policy over the last quarter of a century or so. In many respects, England has led the way internationally in efforts to reduce socioeconomic inequalities in health (Mackenbach, 2010). A comprehensive strategy and series of targets underpinned much of this agenda, especially during the years of Labour government between 1997 and 2010. However, attempts to reduce inequalities in health have been far from uniformly successful. It will be argued here that this is not altogether surprising when we take a broad view of the determinants of health and of the structure of health systems (in the widest possible sense) in England. Consequently, this book will focus on the relationship between health inequalities, theory, policy and practice.

According to Graham the term 'health inequalities' is used to 'describe the systematic differences in health associated with people's different and unequal positions in society. In other words, the concept links the health of individuals to the structures of social inequality which shape their lives' (2004: 117). Furthermore, she emphasises that in most countries, including the UK, health inequalities are often used as shorthand for socioeconomic inequalities in health, whether measured at an individual or an area level (for Graham, health inequalities which relate to other structures of inequality are labelled as, for example, gender or ethnic inequalities in health). The World Health Organization (WHO) Commission on Social Determinants of Health provides a broader holistic and global view of the social determinants of health:

> The poor health of the poor, the social gradient in health within countries, and the marked health inequities between countries are caused by the unequal distribution of power, income, goods, and services, globally and nationally, the consequent unfairness in the immediate, visible circumstances of people's lives – their access to health care, schools, and education, their conditions of work and leisure, their homes, communities, towns, or cities – and their chances of leading a flourishing life. (WHO, 2008: 1)

Health inequalities are complex. They relate to social status and wealth, within and between countries; the quality of, and access to, services within the health sector and other publically funded services; and to the overall quality of life and amenities available to people where they live and work (or importantly, if they are unemployed, don't work). If we accept this view then we must also accept that it has serious implications for the ways in which health inequalities are understood and for the potential approaches to tackling and remedying them. The WHO Commission states that since their roots are embedded in the deep social structures of modern societies, an equally fundamental approach to change is necessary if health inequalities are to be eradicated or at least narrowed:

> In order to address health inequalities, and the inequitable conditions of daily living, it is necessary to address inequalities – such as those between men and women – in the way society is organized. This requires a strong public sector that is committed, capable, and adequately financed. To achieve that requires more than strengthened government – it requires strengthened governance: legitimacy, space, and support for civil society, for an accountable private sector, and for people across society to agree public interests and reinvest in the value of collective action. In a globalized world, the need for governance dedicated to equity applies equally from the community level to global institutions. (WHO, 2008: 2)

Turning this conceptualisation into practice is a complex operation and is contingent on local contexts. Curtis (2008: 299), for example, emphasises that not all elements of civil society are as easy to engage in debates about health, especially those marginal groups who often experience health inequalities most sharply. We shall expand on issues such as this in Chapter Two. However, it is worth noting for now that even with adequate resources and a fair wind supporting a reduction in health inequalities in principle, many issues around the types of action, the governance arrangements for delivering this action and the evidence base for the types of interventions required to reduce health inequalities also need to be resolved. This has implications from international to local levels of action and interaction.

The WHO Commission was followed in England by a strategic review of health inequalities post-2010 called *Fair society, healthy lives*, also led by Professor Michael Marmot. The Marmot Review also developed a view of health inequalities, applied to the English setting, which is strongly associated with the social determinants of health. In other words, as Marmot effectively argues, people's health is related to their social position, and the lower this is the worse their health is likely to be:

> In England, inequalities in health exist across a range of social and demographic indicators, including income, social class, occupation and parental occupation, level of education, housing condition, neighbourhood quality, geographic region, gender and ethnicity. Inequalities are evident in many health outcomes, including mortality, morbidity, self-reported health, mental health, death and injury from accidents and violence. (2010: 45)

The Marmot Review was a detailed strategic review of health inequalities that sought to develop evidence most relevant to underpinning future policy and action. In doing so, the quote above illustrates the extent to which different types of social and demographic conditions can impact on a person's health.

Given this broadly socially determined view of health inequalities, it is necessary to consider what can be done. For example, Sassi (2005: 70) notes that 'there is generally recognition that health disparities are likely to persist as long as social structures allow some degree of inequality'. Furthermore, Scambler (2011) writes that a given population's health, and the differential distribution of health throughout that population, is more a function of the characteristics of a society than it is of a society's health care system. Scambler continues by applying the tension between Burawoy's (2005) 'policy sociology' and 'critical sociology' to health inequalities. He points out that the former is concerned with informing and promoting interventions to tackle health inequalities, while the latter is concerned with contextualising policies and interventions in terms of broader systemic and structural forces. Consequently, there are two ways of broadly defining health inequalities as a research problem.

- Health inequalities can be conceptualised as a policy problem with clear targets that assume it is possible to narrow gaps in health outcomes based on policy action but not fundamental social or economic change. This approach has tended to emphasise local intervention, although often with wider policy measures (that, however, are often not targeted on health improvement as such, but on aspects such as income maintenance and housing improvements).

4

- Health inequalities are 'wicked problems' and are largely intractable in post-industrial capitalist economies like England due to structural factors and social determinants. The argument here goes that we need to change the structure of the economy and society to have a significant impact on health inequalities.

In this book we want to ride both horses. Just because we agree with the second statement does not mean we should not try to address the former and make policy on inequalities per se as effective as possible, as well as trying to address more fundamental societal inequalities. Consequently, both of these themes will be threads running throughout the book.

We are particularly interested in explanations of health inequalities that are informed by complex realism. As a result, we need to be clear from the outset about the ontological and epistemological stance of the book. The approach to how the world may be known (epistemology) depends on the fundamental understanding of what the world actually is (ontology) (Byrne, 2011). For Introna, 'the dominant ontology for social systems is that they are *socially constructed and historically emerging* phenomena' (2003: 209). In this book we draw on critical and complex realism, which views the social world as constituted of complex open systems (see Byrne, 2011 for a fuller account). This approach signals an insistence on 'really existing' generative mechanisms, and acknowledges that the social world is comprised of 'interactions, emergent properties and non-linear changes', with complexity theory a way of framing this (Blackman, 2006: 32). In doing so, we argue that this understanding of the social world is particularly well suited to the nature of health inequalities.

Health inequalities are an issue for which there have been wide variations across the local planning and administrative areas of the National Health Service (NHS) and local government in England in the extent of progress made towards nationally determined targets (DH, 2006; 2007a). Matheson et al point out that differences of this kind can be more fully understood when focusing on the interrelationships of a complex system. That is:

> differences result from the interactions that occur between and among parts of a collective, between and among parts and collectives, and between and among collectives. The theoretical picture this creates is one of overlapping systems that have some coherence but are also linked to, and part

of, other systems that are continually adapting to each other. (2009: 223)

As a consequence of this complexity, health inequalities can be considered to be 'wicked problems' (see, for example, Blackman et al, 2006; Petticrew et al, 2009). Wicked problems are described as complex, difficult to define, lacking an immediate solution and able to be considered a symptom of another problem (Rittel and Webber, 1973). Rittel and Webber contrast these with 'tame' problems: these are not necessarily simple, since they can be very technically complicated, but they can be tightly defined and a solution fairly readily identified and/or walked through (Blackman et al, 2010). Blackman (2006) contends that health inequalities cannot be categorised in these terms: rather, they must be conceptualised as essentially complex phenomena in respect of both their causation and the interventions needed to tackle them. In addition, he emphasises:

> There is growing recognition in policy discourses of the complexity of wicked issues, and the need for changes in local governance to create capacity to intervene in causal combinations, rather than through the traditional silos of public service delivery. There is a challenge here for researchers to match this capacity with useful theory and evidence appropriate to this new governance context. (2006: 54)

We will return to these issues and to the need to devise new strategies to address health inequalities in both policy making and academic fields throughout the book. Nevertheless, it is worth re-emphasising at this stage that health inequalities have many of the characteristics of wicked problems and that the issue sits well with the notion of a social world constituted of complex open systems.

Potential causes

When discussing the causes of health inequalities we must first consider the notion of *causation*. Conventionally, quantitative approaches to causality in social science have in common a focus on the relation between supposedly independent (predictive and/or causal) variables and a dependent outcome variable (Blackman et al, 2011a). Attempts are made to locate the independent average net effect of one variable on another, while controlling for the effects of other independent variables. However, Byrne (2012:18) questions the reality of variables as entities that can be detached from real social cases as the objects of social reality. Variables can be measured, Byrne notes, but they are not entities existing in and of themselves. Furthermore, complex systems have emergent properties that cannot be reduced to component parts; thus, we cannot assign partial contributions to discrete variables (Byrne, 2012: 19).

We will return to this argument in more detail in Chapter Four. It is useful to illustrate this point here, though, by taking premature mortality rates resulting from cancer as an example of health inequalities. Some of the potential causes of this for individuals (as 'cases') relate to a complex combination of lifestyle behaviours such as smoking, diet, exercise, bodyweight and exposure to sunlight. It is very difficult to isolate these behaviours accurately and attribute causation to these as individual variables. Indeed, we can question whether this is a desirable strategy, given that in practice people do not live their lives in neat and separate component parts: diet, frequency of exercise, social and work activities, alcohol and nicotine consumption are all parts of the complex whole that make up individuals' lifestyles. But this is not the whole picture because lifestyle, in turn, relates to (but is not wholly determined by) the contexts in which people live their lives. Different people react to these different contexts differently. When we talk about contexts here we take a multi-scalar approach, including family, workplace, neighbourhood settings, towns, cities and regions – all important contextual characteristics within which people lead their lives. Here we are talking about multiple and non-linear causation in which individuals are embedded and the importance of *interactions* between these multiple causes. It follows that we should take a research approach that concentrates on the interactions between people and settings rather than trying to distinguish between independent health effects of individual characteristics and behaviours (Cummins et al, 2007). The significance of these different approaches to understanding and assessing the causation and impact of health inequalities will be explored in more detail throughout Part One of the book.

Having briefly set out the approach to causation at the core of this book we will now look at some of the wide variety of causes of health inequalities in England that have previously been identified. In doing so, we turn to the findings of the Marmot Review (2010) and, in particular, the second chapter on 'health inequalities and the social determinants of health'. This provides an analysis of the causes, variety and extent of health inequalities in England, which is particularly useful because it has become the basis for contemporary policy on public health, apparently accepted by both the Conservative/Liberal Democrat Coalition government in England and its Labour predecessor.

Following the change of government in 2010, the new administration asserted a continuing commitment to this issue by stating that 'tackling health inequalities and promoting equality is central if the NHS is to deliver health outcomes that are among the best in the world' (DH, 2010a: 4). The subsequent Health and Social Care Bill 2011 proposed a new duty, both nationally and locally, to reduce inequalities, in which:

- 'The Secretary of State must have regard to the need to reduce inequalities between the people of England with respect to the benefits that they can obtain from the health service';
- 'each clinical commissioning group [the local health service commissioning organisations replacing local NHS Primary Care Trusts (PCTs)] must, in the exercise of its functions, have regard to the need to (a) reduce inequalities between patients with respect to their ability to access health services; (b) reduce inequalities between patients with respect to the outcomes achieved for them by the provision of health services';health improvement responsibilities and funding were transferred from PCTs to local government.

The Marmot Review makes clear that the gap in life expectancy between social classes has persisted throughout the period with which it is concerned (1971 to 2005). The second chapter of the Review concentrates on a number of areas of health inequalities, including the English health inequalities targets up to 2010; further indicators of relevance to the social gradient in health; behavioural risk factors for ill health; and the causes of the causes of health inequalities (Marmot, 2010). By focusing on these in some detail below, we intend to highlight the diversity and complexity of health inequalities in terms of both the potential causes and how they manifest themselves in different settings.

The Marmot Review first looks at the English public service agreement (PSA) health inequality target, which was established in 2001 and had two main strands:

- **infant mortality** – a target to reduce by 10% the gap in mortality for children under 1 year old between the 'routine and manual occupation group' and the population as a whole by 2010;
- **life expectancy** – a target to reduce by at least 10% the gap in life expectancy between the fifth of areas with the worst health and deprivation indicators (the 'Spearhead' group of local authorities)

and the population as a whole by 2010. There were also specific sub-targets for reducing relative mortality in heart disease and cancer.

We shall reflect on progress towards these targets in Chapter Six and Part Three of the book. It is worth noting now that these targets relate to different occupational groups and geographical areas. The targets imply the possibility that health inequalities can be purposively reduced between social classes and between, and within, local administrative boundaries. Consequently, interventions to improve health and reduce inequalities were targeted towards particular groups in society and to geographical areas that had poorer health. The types of interventions and the organisations delivering them varied considerably. These differences and their effects (and effectiveness) in different contexts will be considered in detail in Parts Two and Three of the book.

The Marmot Review's next focus is on a number of further indicators of health of relevance to the social gradient in health (2010: 48). First, social gradients in health vary by region, with those in the North West and North East being especially steep. However, managerial and professional classes have similar and lower levels of mortality wherever they live. Long-term illness (morbidity) also follows a social gradient with, for example, those in some of the managerial and professional classes not reaching the same illness rates until they are 65 and over as those aged 45–64 in routine and manual jobs (Marmot, 2010). Cancer and circulatory diseases are often called the 'big killers' in more developed economies, being among the main causes of death in countries like England. The Review identifies social inequalities in these diseases among the more deprived social classes.

The Marmot Review (2010: 52–9) outlines four main behavioural risk factors for ill health.

- **Smoking**. Higher proportions of people in households classified as 'routine and manual' smoke.
- **Alcohol**. While people with lower social economic status are more likely to abstain from alcohol, those that do consume are more likely to have problematic drinking patterns and dependence.
- **Obesity**. In England, like other high-income countries, obesity is associated with social and economic deprivation.
- **Drug use**. There are strong associations between drug use and deprivation in England.

It takes a number of areas as being 'particularly powerful in shaping health and health inequalities' (2010: 60–81). These are called the 'causes of the causes' and the 'social determinants of health' and include the following.

- **Early years**. Social gradients in health begin before birth and increase throughout childhood. Physical, social and cognitive development during the early years of life influence educational attainment, economic participation and health.
- **Education and health**. Socioeconomic deprivation has an adverse impact at each stage of educational development. In addition, there are differences in attainment related to gender and ethnicity.
- **Work, health and wellbeing**. Patterns of employment reflect and reinforce the social gradient and there is inequality of access to labour market opportunities. Insecure and poor-quality employment is associated with an increased risk of physical and mental health worsening.
- **Income and health**. There is a well-established relationship between low income and health with people on low incomes refraining from or being unable to purchase goods and services that maintain or improve health. Also poor health can result in lower earning capacity. Accumulation of wealth through home ownership, working patterns and personal wealth are also important determinants of household wealth and wellbeing.
- **Communities and health**. Attributes listed here include: sustainable communities – people on low incomes are more likely to be affected by risks from climate change such as urban heat islands and less likely to be protected from the risks such as poor housing and access to insurance; social gradients in places and neighbourhoods – the more deprived a neighbourhood, the more likely it is to have social and environmental characteristics presenting risks to health; housing – the poorest groups have become concentrated in both social and poor-quality housing, which can present risks to health; fuel poverty – single pensioners and workless households are more likely to be unable to afford to heat their homes and prevent ill health from cold; and transport – inequalities are apparent in terms of access to opportunities like work, education and social networks, and in terms of higher numbers of road deaths for children from more deprived areas.

Following the identification of the areas in which the social gradient is particularly evident, the Marmot Review concludes this overview by emphasising that:

All the inequalities described in this chapter have persistent and complex causes and relationships are multi-faceted, between, for instance, early years, education, employment, living environment, income and health. A person's physical and mental health is profoundly shaped by their experiences in all these areas and multiple disadvantages compound to produce significantly worse physical and mental health and well-being. (2010: 84)

This conclusion can usefully be read alongside that of the WHO Commission on Social Determinants of Health, which Marmot also led:

This unequal distribution of health-damaging experiences is not in any sense a 'natural' phenomenon but is the result of a toxic combination of poor social policies and programmes, unfair economic arrangements, and bad politics. Together, the structural determinants and conditions of daily life constitute the social determinants of health and are responsible for a major part of health inequalities between and within countries. (WHO, 2008: 1)

This demonstrated why this book needs to, and will, adopt perspectives of critical and not just policy sociology. On the one hand, 'good' policies and practice need to be developed to address health inequalities in local health systems; on the other, broader structural determinants of health must also be addressed to make these local adaptations as effective as possible.

Health inequalities and the public health agenda

Much of the discussion in this chapter has argued that health inequalities have broad and interrelated causes. These are, in turn, linked to the responsibilities of a similarly broad range of organisations. However, it is also important to recognise that much of the health inequalities debate has been situated in a context in which the public health function is seen to be the lead actor or organisation. Hunter et al (2010) note that the public health system in England is contested, with no single or simple definition. They also suggest that 'if it is to succeed, public health needs to adapt to changing contexts and, in doing so, to address a number of long-standing issues that have hitherto hampered the public health function and prevented it from realising its full potential'

(2010: 1). Other commentators have emphasised different stages in the development of public health, in which different characteristics have been particularly prominent. Peckham and Exworthy (2003: 221–2) identify four such stages:

- sanitation, better living spaces, improved working conditions and control of diseases such as cholera and typhoid;
- the shift to preventive medicine in the Victorian period;
- the medicalisation of public health in the twentieth century – a narrow definition focusing on hygiene, epidemiology and disease control; and
- the development of the 'New Public Health' towards the end of the twentieth century and an increasing focus on health promotion, prevention and rehabilitation.[2]

A fundamental aspect of the contested nature of public health highlighted by Curtis (2008), Davis et al (2011) and Wistow (2012), among others, is the tension between medicine and health services managed by the NHS on the one hand, and the wellbeing function of local government on the other. Wistow (2012) identifies two principles that have been fundamental weaknesses of the arrangements between the NHS and local government, and traces the origins of these back to the creation of the NHS and the form of its first major reorganisation in 1974. First, NHS and local government structures were built around the skills of providers rather than the needs of users; second, they sought to privilege internal over external integration through, for example, the transfer of public health from local authorities to the NHS. In this respect, therefore, the services were structured to reflect their separate identities and purposes rather than the needs of individuals and populations for functional integration. We will return to these arrangements and principles in Part Two of the book.

Curtis (2008) has suggested that public health and wellbeing are being reclaimed as legitimate activities for local government. Hunter et al claim that this process is part of a wider set of changes in health systems, whereby 'issues that were previously viewed as distinct and separate are now regarded as inextricably linked through their impact on health' (2010:1). In the 1980s and early 1990s there was a very strong emphasis on individual responsibility for health in the UK, while from the late 1990s there has been a (limited) reorientation towards government policy as a vehicle to address health inequalities, based on collective responsibility to address the wider determinants of health (Curtis, 2008). However, the health inequalities policy stream has a history of being somewhat 'muddy', according to Exworthy and Powell (2004: 270). An example they use is the tension between reducing health inequalities and improving levels of health in the population overall (which may be achieved at the expense of widening inequalities in health between some groups). Other implementation challenges include the long-term nature of the causes of health inequalities and the need for joint working between agencies (such as PCTs and local government) to address them, with their separate budgets and authority. Consequently, Exworthy and Powell (2004: 272) point out that agencies did not focus as much attention on health inequalities as on 'hard' targets such as waiting lists for treatment that were regarded as more important, immediate and individually owned.

Hunter et al argue that 'the notion of a public health system can provide a useful organising device or framework to bring together various sectors, statutory and non-statutory, that contribute to the public's health' (2010: 24). Their vision of such a system, therefore, is a broadly based one, incorporating both many agencies formally responsible for public health (such as the NHS and local government) and those without those responsibilities, such as lobbying and campaigning groups. To these agencies we should also add community and voluntary organisations. Hunter et al (2010: 37) identify the functions of public health as comprising three overlapping domains – health protection, health improvement and health service quality improvement – each of which, to further complicate matters, has a complex system of advisory bodies and arm's length bodies, as well as some areas of shared responsibility.

While this 'public administration' categorisation of the public health function is not without value, we shall approach it and its relationship to the alleviation of health inequalities from a different perspective, namely that of complexity theory and complex realism (Byrne, 2011). More specifically, we follow Teisman et al's (2009) application of complexity theory to governance systems to explore the role of the public health system in tackling health inequalities. In doing so, we adopt the view that interactions in governance networks are complex, with outcomes of interactions the result of both the intentions and actions of agents and 'interferences' from the contexts in which interactions take place.

Plan of the book

Much of the discussion above will be revisited in more detail throughout the book. However, it has been important from the outset to identify and establish our view of health inequalities and how this fits with our view of the world and our approach to understanding it. This book does not claim to resolve issues relating to different evidence bases and academic debates around health inequalities, as well as underlying political differences, since the extent of acceptable health inequality is at heart a political issue. Rather, it argues that the way in which we view the world is significant, and that adopting a critical and complex realist approach is entirely appropriate for an issue such as health inequalities. In doing so, we seek to build on the work of Blackman (2006), Blackman et al (2011a; 2011b) and Byrne (2011) by applying this framing to health inequalities.

The book is divided into three parts. Part One (Chapters Two to Four) is concerned with context and theory, and with developing an applied approach to studying health inequalities. This essentially provides the theoretical framework for what follows, identifying why health inequalities exist and setting out key concepts to guide our approach to understanding them. Part Two (Chapters Five and Six) focuses on health inequalities in England. We consider the history of health inequalities in England, the role of the NHS and the role of local government and other non-NHS partners. Finally, Part Three (Chapters Seven and Eight) considers case studies from the Health Inequalities National Support Team (HINST) and a study of progress towards meeting the health inequalities targets in England that were meant to be achieved by 2010.

Part One: Context and theory: developing an applied approach to studying health inequalities

Chapter Two begins by considering what we mean by 'health' and by 'inequalities'. The chapter is then divided into two broad but related themes that introduce the notion of health inequalities as wicked problems and situate this within discussions about complexity and complex realism. In this respect, Petticrew et al (2009) believe that generating better evidence also means producing more robust evidence, and that the task of collecting evidence about reducing health inequalities through social determinants is especially difficult precisely because it is a wicked problem. Further, interactions in governance systems are complex. Outcomes of interactions are the results of not only the intentions and actions of agents but also the context in which interactions take place (Teisman et al, 2009). Consequently, a key concern of this chapter is how we should research these issues.

Chapter Three outlines a whole system approach to account for the complexities of health inequalities as part of local systems as fully as possible. It builds on research undertaken for a UK National Institute for Health Research-funded project titled 'Comparative analysis of how local system factors affect progress tackling health inequalities'. In outlining the system, an applied approach to health inequalities research is illustrated by focusing, in particular, on the questionnaire and secondary dataset that formed an important part of the study design by framing the issues. The study adopted Wrede et al's (2006) analysis of outcomes being a reflection of the purposeful design of services, the nature of interactions between agents, and contextual attributes. As a result, it is stressed that researching health inequalities outcomes requires a necessarily broad framework for investigation. The chapter is divided into two main sections.

- **Approaches to tackling health inequalities**. The focus here is on approaches to policy and practice and different types of intervention, such as the identification and targeting of health inequalities; the role of commissioning; the role of partnership working; community engagement; the public health workforce; leadership; organisational culture; prioritisation of gaps; and intervention settings. These can all be considered to play an important role in tackling health inequalities.
- **The importance of context**. The discussion draws and expands on issues highlighted by our secondary data collection. The focus is on such conditions as the level of deprivation; housing; 'liveability'; crime rates; PCT budget allocations; PCT star ratings of performance; education attainment; primary care performance data (via the Quality and Outcomes Framework (QOF)); and number of general practitioners (GPs) per head.

Chapter Four provides the reader with an introduction to measurement and causality. This is particularly significant given the targets that were adopted by Labour governments over the 1997–2010 period around health inequalities, and the complexity of the issue for researchers and policy makers to grapple with. It is argued that indicators of health inequalities such as life expectancy can be viewed as outcomes of the dynamic systems that produce them, and that identifying traces of these systems is central to developing an understanding of health inequalities and their causes (Byrne, 2002).

Part Two: Health inequalities in England

Chapter Five offers a historical account of health inequalities in England. It does so by providing a chronological overview of key developments in addressing the causes of health inequalities in England and policy geared towards tackling these. First, we provide an introduction to the early public health movement and how this related to health inequalities. The next section is concerned with health inequalities in England in the period following the Second World War. The development of the NHS and the universalisation of health services are considered in relation to the limited impact these had on reducing health inequalities in England. Next, we move on to consider the Black Report and how this responded to the growing gaps in health between social classes. The chapter then provides an overview of policy following the Black Report, up to and including the Acheson Report in 1998. We then consider in more detail the 1997–2010 Labour period. Particular focus is given to the health inequalities strategy, which set out to reduce the gap in infant mortality across social groups and raise life expectancy faster in the most disadvantaged areas than elsewhere.

Chapter Six considers the changes to the health inequalities policy agenda in England since the Coalition government came to power in May 2010. The chapter begins with an overview of the position around health inequalities in 2010, taking into consideration the findings of the Marmot Review, which provided a significant landmark in the health inequalities field in both assessing and recommending future developments for health inequalities policy and practice in England. We then discuss wider developments in policy that have an important bearing on health inequalities. These include likely implications of the austerity agenda and the 'Big Society' programme for health inequalities. Next, we explore changes to policy and practice instigated by the Coalition government that have relevance for the health inequalities field. These include but are not limited to the new health and social care arrangements put in place under the Health and Social Care Act 2012.

Part Three: Case studies

Part Three of the book provides two detailed case studies focusing on policy and practice around the health inequalities targets established under the New Labour government. The chapter by two members of the Health Inequalities National Support Team (HINST) relates to the work carried out by the team between 2007 and 2011. The qualitative comparative analysis (QCA) case study chapter uses health inequalities data that was available at the time a research project was being conducted by a number of the authors of this book. As such, some of the content of this part of the book is a little out of date, given that HINST was closed down early in the life of the Coalition government, and the research project – which is the focus of Chapter Eight – concluded in 2010. While the results from these chapters relate to a particular period of health inequalities policy and practice, the methods and approaches outlined here have a more general application in terms of conceptualising health inequalities and understanding progress towards narrowing these through systematic, practical action.

Chapter Seven provides a summary of evidence for public health practice derived from the work of HINST. In so doing, the context for and evolution of HINST are discussed. The chapter then provides an overview of the principles that underpinned the HINST approach, including their principles for intervention; approaches to population-level change; and holistic approach to commissioning. This is followed by a number of practical illustrations of effective practice identified by HINST. The chapter concludes with some reflections on the implications for the new policy environment following the election of the Coalition government in 2010. Although the approaches set out in this chapter were designed for systems that have since changed in England, their underlying principles remain and are still of direct interest and are being applied by the organisations that now have responsibility for reducing health inequalities.

Chapter Eight draws on the results of the National Institute for Health Research study highlighted above. It includes an introduction to the case-based research method of QCA as a research approach, linking this to the methodological issues raised in Part One of the book. The results of the study are discussed for three health inequality outcome areas: cancers, cardiovascular disease (CVD) and teenage conceptions. These demonstrate some of the diversity in health inequalities, and the results highlight different 'pathways' to narrowing or widening health gaps.

Conclusions

Chapter Nine focuses on key issues that have emerged in the preceding chapters and on lessons for practice and research. We explore the role of different parts of the NHS in tackling (and potentially enhancing) inequalities in health. Not all measures to improve health are likely to narrow health inequalities, and doing nothing may of itself increase inequalities. For example, access to and use of primary care services can vary considerably by social class. In the exploration we make connections between earlier discussions about public health and how these link to the broader governance of health inequalities across a plurality of providers from a range of non–NHS organisations to community and voluntary sector groups. Together, these form a fluid and permeable public health system. This, in turn, relates to a central theme of the book, namely the complexity of health inequalities, and we conclude our discussion by reflecting on the methodological and practical implications of delivering and implementing policies for such a complex issue in terms of both its conceptualisation and the often fragmented mechanisms that are employed to reduce health inequalities.

Part One
Context and theory: developing an applied approach to studying health inequalities

---

TWO

Health inequalities, wicked problems and complexity

Introduction

We have already noted that the term 'health inequalities' is used to describe systematic differences in health status between, and within, different socioeconomic groups. We've also recognised that the social (including economic) determinants of health are broad and complex. Before considering the development of policy responses in England in relation to health inequalities, it will be useful to understand better the concepts of health and inequality. This analysis forms part of the context for understanding the nature of policy options and outcomes. To do so, as noted in the previous chapter, we need to consider the notions of complexity and wicked problems more fully. Together, these concepts provide fundamental underpinnings of the perspective adopted in this book to help understand the nature of health, health inequalities and possible strategies for addressing them. Consequently, this chapter provides our approach to framing and making sense of health inequalities.

What is health?

> 'The whole point of this country is if you want to eat garbage, balloon up to 600lbs, and die of a heart attack at 43, you can. You are free to do so. To me that is beautiful.'
> (Ron Swanson,[3] Parks and Recreation, NBC [National Broadcasting Company])

Ron Swanson has a point. In terms of our lifestyles and health-related behaviours we have wide areas of discretion. Like him, we also recognise that these freedoms do not necessarily lead to good health outcomes for us as individuals or (as he fails to add) for society and the state more widely. Moreover, the extent and exercise of such discretionary health-related behaviours are neither unbounded nor random. So-called free choice is a chimera.[4] Both it and our linked behaviours are socially and economically structured by many influences in our different environments. We have noted in the previous chapter that the social gradient is a key determinant of health inequalities and their associated outcomes. We can begin to deepen our understanding of the relationship between social inequality and health status as we explore more closely what we mean by health.

The constitution of the World Health Organization (WHO) defines health as 'a state of complete physical, mental and social well-being and not merely the absence of disease or infirmity' (WHO, 1948). For Illich (1976: 7), on the other hand, 'health' is an everyday word used 'to designate the intensity with which individuals cope with their internal states and environmental conditions'. He also argues that the health of populations depends on the way in which political actions create the environment and circumstances that favour self-reliance, dignity and autonomy for all. Taylor and Marandi (2008) state that 'social determinants – social, economic, political, cultural, and environmental factors – heavily influence people's demand for, access to, and use of health services'. In other words, social determinants cut across why and how people become ill, and how – and whether – they are treated by health and health-related professionals. What all these viewpoints have in common is a fundamental understanding of health as being socially structured and not merely to be equated with the absence of remediable disease or the treatment of ill health. In short, we can expect to find social as well as medical models of causation and intervention in the broad field of health. The topic of disability provides a very clear example of differences in conceptions of health.

Models of health

In 1983 Mike Oliver conceptualised models of disability through a binary distinction between individual and social models of disability. For Oliver, the individual model is underpinned by what he calls the 'personal tragedy' theory of disability which, in turn, is underpinned by the medical model of health. From this perspective, the condition of the 'disabled', their 'limitations' and 'problems' are the consequence of an individual characteristic:

> I locate the medicalisation of disability within the individual model and as I have argued that this model is inappropriate, so, it logically follows, is the medicalisation process ... disability is a social state and not a medical condition. Hence medical intervention in, and more importantly, control over

> disability is inappropriate. Doctors are trained to diagnose, treat and cure illnesses, not to alleviate social conditions or circumstances. (Oliver, 1990: 3)

The social model of disability does not deny the 'problem' of disability but locates it squarely within society. It is not individual limitations which are the cause of the problem but society's failure to provide appropriate services and adequately ensure that the needs of disabled people are fully taken into account in its social organisation. This is a powerful argument, which has great resonance for how we choose to view health more generally and inequalities in health in particular. How far do we understand inequalities in health outcomes as a problem of the individuals experiencing them or as a product of, and problem for, society? We are explicitly formulating our concern in these terms to avoid polarising the medical and social models of health too sharply. Rather, we wish to explore the case for rebalancing the medical and social models. It is a distinction, therefore, that provides a framework within which both to identify and to consider the balance between different approaches for improving health and reducing health inequalities. We use it in the remainder of this section as we turn to the role of two key strategies frequently advocated for improving the health of individuals and populations: health promotion and health services delivery.

The role of health promotion

If we adopt an understanding of health as being socially determined, the role of health promotion cannot be restricted to the modification of individual behaviours. If, at the same time, we also recognise that the social determinants of health lie largely outside the role and influence of health services, it follows that health promotion is necessarily conceptually complex and organisationally complicated (Baum, 2007). Warr et al reflect this understanding in arguing that 'health promotion is the process of enabling people to increase control over, and to improve, their health. It moves beyond a focus on individual behaviour towards a wide range of social and environmental interventions' (2013: 95). In their study of health promotion in Australia, the same authors suggest that the field is characterised by two categories of activity: 'procedural' and 'cooperative'. The former is a specialised set of activities and technical knowledge focused on the dissemination of health information, while the latter comprises a broader-based approach focused on socioeconomic and health equality and delivered through processes of community engagement and participation as well as professional service delivery systems. As a result, they suggest, health promotion workers in community-based contexts must move between two radically different ways of working (the cooperative and procedural) so as to navigate the frequently conflicting demands of community, service and professional expectations (Warr et al, 2013: 106). Indeed, they suggest there may even be a direct conflict between the growing professionalisation of health promotion and its delivery on the one hand, and its ability to stimulate collective community action approaches to address socioeconomic disadvantage on the other (Warr et al, 2013: 107). Whatever the case, it is clear that a service model based on providing information to individuals so that they are better equipped to maintain and improve their own health calls on different skills and understandings from one which seeks to address the social determinants of health through collective social action. Both approaches may have important roles to play but, if we accept our earlier point that health-promoting choices and behaviours are socially structured, the provision of information alone is unlikely to overcome the influence of social determinants and may even reinforce their impact.

Impact of social determinants

The impact of social determinants is not absent from the related field of the early detection and treatment of disease (which is more closely related to the individual/medical model of health). Social determinants affect not only the distribution of disease but also the distribution of and access to services intended to be part of the National Health Service (NHS)'s supposedly universal offer of care and treatment. As Dorling (2013a: 11) demonstrates, high levels of economic inequality may push medical practitioners away from those most in need. By this he means that medical doctors prefer to live and work in the areas of higher socioeconomic status in which better health outcomes are concentrated. In more equitable countries, doctors tend not to avoid serving areas with greater health needs because the differences are less pronounced (Dorling, 2013a). Evidence for the existence of an 'inverse care law' (Tudor Hart, 1971), according to which services are distributed inversely to population health needs,[5] has been repeatedly demonstrated in the UK: people living in areas where need is relatively low have better access to the most specialised and skilled medical services (Shaw and Dorling, 2004). By contrast, the same authors derived data from the 2001 census, which apparently demonstrates that informal care (provided by the families and friends of those in need and at limited extra cost to the state save the benefits and allowances paid to some carers) is provided in almost direct and exact proportion to need. This conclusion led Shaw and Dorling (2004) to postulate the operation of a 'positive care law' in relation to informal care, where the cheapest (for the state) and least skilled form of care is positively related to need. We also need to recognise that informal care may also be what people need and families want to see supplied as part of an agreed mix of formal and informal services. For example, Wistow et al (2015) found that during emergencies older people tend to turn to informal networks of care in the first instance, and out of preference, rather than more formal networks.

Whether we take a narrower (individual/medical) or broader (social) view of health, there are clear disadvantages in terms of health outcomes for those occupying lower socioeconomic positions. At the same time, Kelly points out that:

> a fully-rounded approach to public health requires both the individual and social levels of explanation … to capture the significant interactions between the individual and social level phenomena. These interactions are important because they not only articulate the causal pathways to the individual disease outcomes, but they demonstrate the various linkages between different phenomena. (2010: 271)

An understanding of these linkages is fundamental to the design of appropriate interventions. In this respect, Taylor and Marandi argue that '[health inequity] is not inevitable. Health care systems and services can promote health equity if they are designed to maximise the "fit" between patients' needs and providers' supply' (2008: 266). Nevertheless, Graham and Kelly (2004) identify that policies aimed at tackling the determinants of health do not automatically tackle the determinants of health inequalities. Instead, we need to focus on the *unequal distribution* of health determinants. In summary, therefore, policy and practice need to recognise that, as Glasby notes, 'people do not start equal and so treating everyone in the same way can perpetuate or exacerbate existing inequalities' (2012: 119). These inequalities are the focus of the next section.

Inequality

Having explored some of the different ways of viewing health, it is also necessary to unpack the notion of inequality further. Inequality is frequently used as a term to describe differences in income between different parts of the population (Cribb et al, 2013). The way we view or interpret different degrees of income inequality tends to be associated with different political and ideological positions. Byrne (2005) identifies three such positions: possessive individualist; liberal 'collectivist'; and Marxist, each of which we briefly consider below. Possessive individuals[6] (originating from Locke's ideas around individual emancipation) view the market as the epitome of rationality, in which citizenship is constructed around individual (as opposed to collective) rights. According to this view, inequality is a natural function of individuals' merits and contributions to society. Liberal collectivists cover a broad church, with the common goal of regulating capitalism in order to ameliorate the excesses of inequality. For traditional Conservatives, the management of capitalism is necessary for maintaining stability in an inherently unstable system. Keynesians, for example, believe in a capitalist system but with progressive taxation to limit economic inequalities. In this view, overall inequality is necessary because the growth of the economy makes us all wealthier. Marxists and socialists regard inequality as essentially exploitative; they want to minimise economic inequality and distribute resources based on individual needs through a project of collective transformation. These different ideological positions have significant implications for the nature of the macroeconomic environments, social structures, local systems and individual lifestyles that will be possible or predominant at any point in time. In England, for example, all of these attributes have been affected in recent years by what is generally accepted to have been a significant shift from socialist collectivism to classic liberalism, explicitly endorsed by almost all political elites in the name of a perceived necessity for a more flexible labour market in a competitive globalised world (Byrne, 2005).

How we view inequality also depends to a large extent on how we view equality. Westergaard and Resler (1975: 281) note that 'equality' is associated with different meanings in America and Europe. In the US the notion of 'equality of opportunity' has been the dominant position, in which each individual will find their own level in the hierarchy of inequality, according to their ability and motivation, and regardless of parentage and the circumstances of early life. The authors point out that there is no challenge to the existence of a socioeconomic hierarchy in itself. The European conception of equality, however, includes just such a challenge in its advocacy of 'equality of condition' and the eradication of significant divisions of power, wealth and security. In reality, Westergaard and Resler (1975) contend, the notion of equality of condition was not generally transferred to policy when social democrats were in office but provided an important buffer to prevent the total encapsulation of labour policies under capitalism.

Inequality and liberal capitalism

Over the past 30–40 years the UK has been a particularly enthusiastic advocate of a free-market form of liberal capitalism. Indeed, Hutton (2003) points out that Blair and Brown were no less enthusiastic about US economic dynamism than Thatcher, and that as result Britain defined itself in Europe as the English-speaking Anglo-Saxon model – a stock market-based capitalism, complete with a minimal welfare system[7] and flexible labour markets. Consequently, the dominant view of inequality has shifted to one of possessive individualists and the view of equality is more closely associated with equality of opportunity. This raises important questions about equity and fairness and whether equality of opportunity can be achieved from an unequal playing field. Key concepts such as social mobility (see Blanden et al, 2005; Goldthorpe and Jackson, 2007), social capital (see Putman, 1995; Ferragina, 2010) and accumulated capital (see Bourdieu, 1986), in particular, draw attention to the significance of social determinants such as social class, family background, ethnicity and geography for environmental inequalities that shape life courses in such a competitive society as that favoured by possessive individualists. This is beyond the strict scope of this book but is highly relevant to our concern with inequalities in health and the extent to which governments are able or wish to influence them. Recognising that successive governments have made ideological choices to pursue a more or less free market-based capitalism, with its implications for socioeconomic inequalities, helps us to understand the context for policy and practice regarding health inequalities and how it has changed over time.

Over the past three decades, for example, wage gaps have increased more in the UK than in most other developed countries (National Equality Panel, 2010). In terms of inequality, Cribb et al (2013) highlight that during the 1960s and 1970s the Gini coefficient[8] fluctuated around 0.26, but during the 1980s it increased substantially, reaching 0.34 by 1990. This was the largest increase in income inequality seen in recent British history and was larger than the rise that took place in other countries at the same time. In the latest figures for 2011–12 the Gini stood at 0.34, which is lower than the pre-recession high of

0.36 in 2007–8 but still significantly higher than in previous decades (Cribb et al, 2013). Rowlingson (2011) suggests that inequality may be particularly harmful after it reaches a particular threshold (0.3 Gini coefficient) and that Britain rose past this in 1986–7. Furthermore, she argues that there is evidence of a correlation between income inequality and health and social problems, and that there is a social gradient in health that means every step up the socioeconomic ladder leads to an increase in health (although it is less clear whether every step up the ladder improves health to the same degree).

The case for greater equality

According to Sassi:

> the evidence would appear to strongly support the case for redistributive policies, and for policies to fight poverty, in a country like the UK. This would not just improve the health of the worse off, and likely reduce health inequalities, but it would also improve overall population health. (2005: 69)

However, he also claims that redistribution tends to have an opportunity cost of reduced growth and average income in the long term, while health policy measures to improve the health of the worse off (economically) tend to require disproportionately large investments. Indeed, Hunter et al note that in England 'part of the difficulty lies in the fact that, while health status is improved across all groups, it is improving at a faster rate in the most advantaged groups, resulting in the health inequalities gap continuing to widen' (2010: 156–7). There is also widespread evidence (as we have already noted and will revisit more fully in Part Two of the book) that access to and use of services in health systems reflect wider social inequalities and tend to favour the better off, sustaining and sometimes amplifying inequalities in health status (Taylor and Marandi, 2008: 266). Consequently, Graham and Kelly argue:

> where health equity is the goal, the priority of a determinants–oriented strategy is to reduce inequalities in the major influences on people's health. Tackling inequalities in social position is likely to be at the heart of such a strategy. It is the pivotal point in the causal chain linking broader ('wider') determinants to the risk factors that directly damage people's health. (2004: 5)

To this end, they suggest a continuum of meanings and strategies for tackling health inequalities: improving the poor health of poor people; narrowing health gaps by raising the health of the poorest fastest; and reducing health gradients so that the standards of health enjoyed by the best off should be attainable by all. It is worth underlining that these strategies are seen as complementary rather than alternative approaches to dealing with health inequalities.

A further trend associated with inequality of health outcomes/status is that of a growing polarisation between the best and worst off in society. Wacquant (2008) associates its development with the growing internal instability of waged work in flexible labour markets. He points out that these have become heterogeneous, differentiated and differentiating, and have moved from being the fount of homogeneity, solidarity and security into a source of social fragmentation and precariousness for those confined to the border zones of the employment sphere. Lee et al focus on this trend in the UK:

> There is concern about wage inequality and employment polarisation the tendency for employment to polarise into low and high skilled work in the UK. Over the long term, the UK labour market has become increasingly polarised into high and low wage employment, and wage inequality has also increased. This is now seen as having harmful social consequences such as potentially reducing social mobility. (2013: 3)

A prominent example of flexible low-wage employment at the time of writing (and potentially subject to new legislation) is the proliferation of 'zero-hours' contracts in the UK. Goodley and Inman (2013) highlight that up to 1 million people in the UK are employed on zero-hours contracts, which offer no guarantee of work or holiday and sick pay. These contracts offer flexibility to employers. However, there are legitimate concerns about the impact of these kinds of contracts on employees. First, the low wages generally associated with this type of contract are likely to intensify the social gradients on health. Rowlingson identifies 'status anxiety' as the most plausible explanation for income inequality's apparent effect on health and social problems. She asserts that 'this suggests that income inequality is harmful because it places people in a hierarchy that increases status competition and causes stress, which leads to poor health and other negative outcomes' (Rowlingson, 2011: 5). Second, the inherent uncertainty and insecurity associated with zero-hours contracts can also be perceived as a threat to health status and wellbeing. The impact on health of such factors is consistent with Marmot's (2004) finding that perceptions of control over individuals' lives are among the most important social determinants of health.

Wicked problems

Health inequalities are often considered to be wicked problems (Blackman, 2006; Blackman et al, 2006; Australian Public Service Commission, 2007; Petticrew et al, 2009). These are issues that are complex in terms of causal pathways, difficult to define and with no immediate solution, with one wicked problem often a symptom of another. In coining the phrase 'wicked problems', Rittel and Webber (1973) argue that there is a whole realm of social planning problems that cannot be successfully tackled with traditional linear, analytical approaches. In calling these 'wicked' they contrast them with 'tame' problems. Blackman et al summarise the differences between wicked and tame problems in Table 2.1.

Table 2.1: Wicked and tame problems

Wicked problem	Tame problem
No definite formulation	Well-defined and stable
Continually evolves and mutates	It is known when a solution is reached
Solutions are better or worse	Solutions are clearly right or wrong
No principles of solution that fit all members of a class of problems	Belongs to a class of similar problems that can be solved in a similar way
Many causal levels, with problems symptoms of other problems	Causes are evident, with solutions that can be tried and abandoned

Source: Blackman et al, 2006: 70.

Tame problems are not necessarily simple, since they can be very technically complicated. However, tame problems can be neatly categorised and solutions are generally easy to identify or work out (Blackman et al, 2010). This is not the case with health inequalities, which should be conceptualised as complex, both with regard to their nature and the actions needed to tackle them (Blackman, 2006).

We develop Blackman et al's (2006) summary of wicked problems in Table 2.1 by directly relating each of the dimensions to health inequalities.

- **No definite formulation**. In Chapter One we used Graham's (2004) definition of health inequalities, which links people's health to unequal positions in society. When we begin to consider this as an issue for policy and/or practice intervention, finding a definitive formulation that can be operationalised widely quickly becomes a complicated challenge. Health inequalities exist within and between localities, the causes and symptoms are highly interrelated and the causal pathways complex, passing through many sectors, including housing, crime, health, social care, welfare and education (Petticrew et al, 2009). Each locality has its own history of socioeconomic development that will affect the nature, and extent, of health inequalities. For example, areas in the north of England have undergone significant levels of deindustrialisation in the past 30–40 years. How localities have responded to a decline in what was once their traditional manufacturing base has had potentially major impacts on the types of communities and neighbourhoods that exist today. Local agencies must take into account these complex local trajectories to formulate effective responses to associated health inequalities. In so doing, expertise needs to be combined across different professional disciplines, often with quite different world views. Consequently, the definition of health inequalities is dependent on time and place, and will often be contested between local community groups and professional bodies.

- **Continually evolves and mutates**. Chapter Five will provide a more detailed discussion of the evolving nature of health inequalities in England. Among others, Dorling (2013a) has charted the historical persistence of health inequalities since the nineteenth century. However, this persistence does not mean that the nature of health inequalities has remained constant over time. For example, in the nineteenth century health inequalities existed through mortality and injuries resulting from poor working conditions in manufacturing industries; by the late twentieth century the focus had shifted to inequalities in what became known as the 'big killers' – cancers and cardiovascular disease. More recently (see Dorling, 2013a) there has been an increasing focus on mortality from road deaths. Furthermore, Green (2013) argues that the processes creating and maintaining health inequalities vary across social, individual and geographic factors and can also be observed through measuring inequalities by age. He also notes that health inequalities are not consistent throughout the life course: 'levels of inequality vary in strength by age and do not always follow traditional social gradients' (2013: 93).

- **Solutions are better or worse rather than right or wrong**. As we have already seen, the Marmot Review identified smoking among households classified as 'routine and manual' to be a key behavioural risk factor in relation to health inequalities. Policy solutions for this were motivated by a national target in England to reduce the rate of smoking by manual workers. Smoking cessation services were a key local policy instrument for tackling this form of inequality. All areas provide this service but the level of provision could, for example, vary in the extent to which they were successful in encouraging general practitioners (GPs) and nurses to refer people to these services; prevalence data was used to target resources; and health equity audits of services had been done. Consequently, this type of solution is unlikely to be right or wrong, but it will have better or worse consequences in particular contexts. A further complicating factor here is the role of targets in performance-management systems. By focusing on four-week quit rates, the smoking cessation target was subject to 'gaming' among local policy makers. In particular, Bevan and Hood (2006) suggest that governance by targets and performance indicators leads to 'output distortions' because it can lead to situations where it appears that only what is measured is what counts. In these circumstances, policy makers and practitioners may be tempted to focus predominantly on ensuring that people stop smoking for a four-week period, rather than whether their interventions are more likely to achieve the harder target of helping them to continue to be non-smokers throughout the remainder of their lives.

- **No principles of solution that fit all members of a class of problems**. Continuing the example of smoking cessation services targeting interventions to reduce health inequalities we should consider whether all smokers are the same. Obviously they are not. Some smokers are more addicted than others; some may identify themselves much more strongly as a 'smoker' than others (it is who they are, rather than something they do); some may be going through a particular difficult period in their life and rely on smoking to manage their mood more than they normally would; for some it may be a key behaviour within a particular social network; and some may be far less concerned[9] about dying prematurely from smoking-related diseases than other smokers. This complexity means that not only is monitoring the smoking status of patients and the public very important; monitoring advice and the response to advice from smoking cessation services is also central to developing solutions to match the diversity of types of need. The role of context and

32

in particular *place* also needs to be considered, as solutions may be better or worse in different settings.

- **Many causal levels, with problems symptoms of other problems**. Curtis argues that while health outcomes are manifested at the local level, at least some of the processes that produce these effects are operating at a wider scale and are subject to regional, national and international processes. Consequently, the effects of, for example, air pollution, climate change, tobacco and alcohol processes, housing and labour markets are subject to these wider processes; these may override any effects of local initiatives to tackle local health conditions and health inequalities (Curtis, 2008: 300).

The application, above, of health inequalities to wicked problems is far from exhaustive. Rather, the intention is to focus on some aspects of health inequalities to illustrate that they are wicked problems. One implication of this, identified by the Australian Public Service Commission, is that as health inequalities are wicked problems they can pose challenges to traditional approaches to policy making and programme implementation:

> Usually, part of the solution to wicked problems involves changing the behaviour of groups of citizens or all citizens. Other key ingredients in solving or at least managing complex policy problems include successfully working across both internal and external organisational boundaries and engaging citizens and stakeholders in policy making and implementation. Wicked problems require innovative, comprehensive solutions that can be modified in the light of experience and on-the-ground feedback. (Australian Public Service Commission, 2007: 2)

It is essential to select methodological approach(es) capable of dealing with such complex contexts and uncertain causal pathways. From this perspective, the necessary characteristic required of an appropriate method for studying wicked problems is the ability to understand causal relationships in complex settings. Klijn (2008: 314) notes that the conceptual framework of complexity theory (a conceptual approach that focuses on the analysis of complex processes and problems) is suitable for so-called wicked problems. The next section will expand on the notion of complexity; however, it is worth noting here the similarities between complexity and wicked problems. Rosen's (1987:

324) distinction between simple and complex systems illustrates this
well:

> a simple system is one to which a notion of state can
> be assigned once and for all, or more generally, one in
> which Aristotlean causal categories can be independently
> segregated from one another. Any system for which such
> a description cannot be provided I will call complex.
> Thus, in a complex system, the causal categories become
> intertwined in such a way that no dualistic language of state
> plus dynamic laws can completely describe it. (quoted in
> Uprichard and Byrne, 2006: 665)

Consequently, when we study health inequalities – and in particular the
causes of these – we need to consider whether it is possible to explain
them as simple systems comprising individual parts, operating within
clearly defined boundaries. The argument above suggests that health
inequalities are not simple. As a result we must turn to complexity.

Complexity

> Some of the great works of art and science are simply beyond
> our comprehension. One of the most beautiful aspects of
> complexity is that it provides us with a description of how
> such things are possible without referring to something
> supernatural. (Cilliers, 2008: 29)

Complexity theory is an interdisciplinary field that has its origins in the
natural sciences. Mitchell (2011: 4) states that a common focus across
academic disciplines is a concern with seeking to explain how large
numbers of relatively simple entities organise themselves, without the
benefit of any central controller, into a collective whole that creates
patterns, uses information and in some cases evolves and learns.
Fundamentally, these approaches attempt to understand change and
the dynamics of systems as a result of the complex interaction of the
parts of those systems (MacIntosh et al, 2006). A common example
of complex systems is ant colonies. These can consist of hundreds
to millions of individual ants, which are simple creatures that work
together to produce complex structures that are of great importance
to the colony as a whole and are much greater than the sum of their
parts (Mitchell, 2011: 4–5).

While complexity theory traditionally focused on physical systems, the social sciences have more recently incorporated constructivist methodology to analyse the actions of agents and subsystems in complex social systems (Teisman et al, 2009). Social science theory has sought to take account of increased complexity, with policy-oriented work particularly concerned with how interventions work across heterogeneous contexts (Pawson and Tilley, 1997; Byrne, 1998; Cilliers, 1998; Wright, 2001). Policy makers have similarly struggled to find solutions to complex problems such as health inequalities that will work predictably in different settings (Griffin, 2006; Kamarck, 2007; Seddon, 2008). However, a number of authors (such as Turner, 1948; Meehl, 1970; Lieberson, 1985; Abbott, 2001) contend that many of the methods used in social science are not well suited to analysing the complex causal patterns that characterise highly differentiated contexts. The nature of such contexts led Cohn et al to argue that 'complexity needs to be understood as a dynamic, ecological system rather than a stable, albeit complicated, arrangement of individual elements' (2013: 40). However, this approach is not one that commonly informs health-related research in England.

Complexity and health research

In March 2009 the House of Commons Health Committee reported on its inquiry into health inequalities, claiming that:

> one of the major difficulties which has beset this inquiry, and indeed is holding back all those involved in trying to tackle health inequalities, is that it is nearly impossible to know what to do given the scarcity of good evidence and good evaluation of current policy. (2009: 5)

However, the Committee's delineation of what should constitute the evidence base for health inequalities reflected a particular view of what comprises good evidence and, specifically, was based on the application of experimental methods to complex social settings. The Committee concluded that simple changes to the design of policy interventions could make all the difference and recommended that future initiatives adhere to a basic set of research guidelines, including piloting, randomisation, controls and the use of quasi-experimental methods where randomisation would be too costly. Blackman et al (2013) note that this approach reflects a particular view among the Committee's politicians (heavily influenced by dominant discourse in medical research) that the best evidence is generated by controlled experiments with random allocation. This takes its place in what has become known as a 'hierarchy of evidence', as outlined in Table 2.2. Kelly (2010: 269) argues that in this hierarchy of evidence the types of study that are capable of understanding the dynamic and relational factors involved in the wider determinants of health are not amenable to data manipulation at the level of meta-analyses or randomised control trials (RCTs).

Table 2.2: Hierarchy of evidence

Hierarchy	Type of evidence
Type I	At least one good systematic review, including at least one RCT
Type II	At least one good RCT
Type III	At least one well-designed intervention study without randomisation
Type IV	At least one well-designed observational study
Type V	Expert opinion, including the views of service users and carers

Source: DH, 1999

In 2000 Medical Research Council (MRC) guidance was ground-breaking in its acknowledgement that many novel health interventions did not consist of singular elements (MRC, 2000). Thus, rather than merely isolating and assessing the efficacy of one component over another, researchers were being asked to evaluate components across different domains all at work simultaneously. However, Cohn et al (2013) point out that this and the MRC guidance that followed it, *Developing and evaluating complex interventions: New guidance* (MRC, 2008), produced an essentially mechanical view of complexity by emphasising that these components are measured as discrete elements, rather than as elements of a dynamic and integrated system. Consequently, for them, the guidance is based on a misunderstanding of complexity.

It is also important to recognise that the ontology and, by implication, epistemology of experimental methods have strongly influenced how evidence is filtered by literature reviews. For example, Dixon-Woods et al state that the:

> Cochrane movement has promoted a hugely influential methodology that might be termed the 'rationalist' model of systematic review. This focuses exclusively on questions concerned with effectiveness, and almost exclusively on

RCTs as means of answering the question of whether something 'works'. (2006: 29)

They write that the advantage of systematic reviews is seen to lie in their rigour and transparency of process, but that they have been increasingly criticised for excluding non-experimental forms of evidence. Petticrew and Roberts (2003: 528) similarly argue against the hierarchy of evidence commonly adopted in systematic reviews, in which the apparent certainty of RCTs is adopted as a 'gold standard' against which all other forms of evidence are measured. In effect, systematic reviews tend to disregard the issue of methodological aptness: different types of research question are best answered by different types of study.[10] Petticrew et al (2009) add that the ability of systematic reviews to inform broader policy and planning needs has not yet been fully realised, in part because it may be difficult to apply their findings, given missing contextual information (a major problem with many RCTs). Above all, this is an argument for explanations that do not focus on simple causation alone (Byrne et al, 2009).

Social theorists tend to view complexity in terms of links between the individual and society, or the behaviour of groups versus individuals, and such behaviours are not reducible to their parts. Cohn et al (2013) contend that capturing more 'sensitive' and sophisticated data (even through the use of mixed methods) is not sufficient: we need to begin by recognising the sheer range of relevant factors and the significance of the variability of local conditions. By seeking to isolate measurable parts (as the MRC guidelines do) we are sacrificing any genuine commitment to complexity. Instead, they go on, we must find a way of understanding the dynamic variability of complexity: 'in other words, the challenge is how to go about studying complexity *without* fully unravelling it' (Cohn et al, 2013: 42). Similarly, Cilliers points out that it is important to consider the limits of our understanding of complex systems and what we can say about them: 'we cannot know a complex system in all its complexity and we, therefore, need to be somewhat modest in our claims about a complex world' (2008: 30).

These claims by Cohn et al and Cilliers raise fundamental questions about the extent to which it is possible to understand the social world in which wicked problems such as health inequalities are located. However, critical realism has developed to provide an ontology and epistemology for addressing this challenge. Critical realism shares with complexity theory an assumption of ontological depth (the notion of social systems as interlinked levels, emerging from, but not reducible to, each other) (Walby et al, 2012: 228). In addition, Bhaskar (1997) has highlighted a related problem that, in the real world, the absence of controlled conditions can undermine causal accounts. Walby et al state that complexity 'helps to avoid the temptation of reductionism either to the micro level of agency or to the macro level of structure; allowing both their place in the analysis' (2012: 228). Similarly, Callaghan (2008: 401) argues that when complexity theory is applied to the social sciences it provides an epistemology for understanding the interactions between structures and human agents. Social systems are reflexive: they are, to a greater or lesser extent, aware of their own historical being – they are self-conscious.

> Their history provides structural constraints on the possibilities open to them. It is precisely the interplay between structure (values, beliefs, predispositions, traditions, language, and existing collaborative practices) and agency (reflexive awareness and interventions) that constitutes and reconstitutes social systems. (Introna, 2003: 210)

A clear implication of this approach is the need to understand systems and their boundaries, an issue to which we now turn.

Scales and boundaries

Matheson et al note that as societies become more interconnected there is a greater need to 'understand the processes of complexity in order to gain insight into the causes of the emergent social patterns – such as health inequalities' (2009: 222). Cilliers (2001), Introna (2003) and Gerrits (2008) all argue that for systems to be recognisable they must have boundaries that set them apart from other systems and/or their environment. However, they also claim that as complex adaptive systems are open, the decision of what is and is not included in these systems is debatable. Cilliers provides a useful definition that describes boundaries as 'something that *constitutes* that which is bounded', rather than something that separates one thing from another (2001: 141). Consequently, boundaries can be viewed as somewhat fuzzy and overlapping but nonetheless useful for characterising social systems. In this section we focus on how to characterise boundaries of complex systems that are of relevance to understanding health inequalities. Three such characteristics are discussed below: organisational arrangements, policy and targets, and place. Each shares a common focus on the relationships between systems and their environments.

Castelli et al (2013) identify an interest in knowing where to best target policies in order to improve health and wellbeing, and in exploring the scope for organisations to exert an influence outside their direct jurisdiction. Key interests can be targeted at the individual, neighbourhood, community, locality, local authority, district, regional or national level. However, it needs to be recognised that the identity of organisations does not, and cannot, remain static (Cilliers, 2001). A study by Barnes et al (2003) illustrates some of the difficulties in identifying the boundaries of organisational arrangements in the field of health inequalities, in relation to health action zones (HAZs) in England. HAZs were a policy initiative under the New Labour government that were designed to improve health and reduce health inequalities, not least through achieving better collaboration across a range of local partners and community groups. Significantly, from our perspective here, Barnes et al found that 'one of the dimensions of HAZ complexity was the way in which it proved impossible to define clearly where "the HAZ" began and ended, what constituted "context" and what constituted the "programme"' (2003: 276). Thus, they point out, context is both part of complex open systems and is subject to change as a result of actions beyond the scope of programmes within the system but also from intended and unintended consequences of programme implementation (Barnes et al, 2003). In addition, this same study showed that what constituted the HAZ was perceived differently by different players, depending in part on their relationship to it. Similarly, a study of health inequalities in New Zealand concluded that when a case incorporates numbers of diverse individuals and social groupings, the framing of a case becomes less immediately apparent (Matheson et al, 2009).

Another way of conceptualising a health inequalities system is to focus on a particular policy target at a local authority administrative level. This approach is a convenient but not entirely unproblematic way to 'bound' a system, given that its boundaries are contingent upon how the relevant target is defined and constituted. This caveat is especially significant in the study of health inequalities targets in England, since targets have been expressed in many different ways, including reductions in infant mortality and increases in life expectancy, together with 12 other headline indicators relating to specific fields. Despite differences between them, the conceptualisation of a system around each target helps to frame an approach that cuts across organisational boundaries and provides a potential basis for joined-up action. It is possible in this respect to consider the targets as addressed by a local system: the network of local agents who come together and are interconnected to fulfil a purpose (Plsek, 2001). Outcomes from this system are a reflection of the purposeful design of services, the nature of interactions between agents, and contextual conditions (Wrede et al, 2006). For example, services may be reactive or proactive; interactions between agents may be more or less aligned to common goals; and contextual conditions such as organisational leadership, aspirations and demographic, ethnic and socioeconomic factors may have a wide range of states. The need to take a whole system perspective follows (and is the focus of Chapter Three). Notwithstanding these potential advantages, we should recognise that perspectives bounded by targets can also have downsides. Among other things, as Bevan and Hood (2006) argue, targets are likely to provide an incomplete and inaccurate picture. In particular, they may lead to systems boundaries being drawn too tightly around the target, with the result that wider determinants of outcomes are neglected.

Methodologically, Buijs et al (2009: 53) claim, we need to move away from traditional public administration (focusing on governmental actors and highly planned and coordinated forms of decision making) to researching particular geographical areas and analysing decisions made here at various arenas and scales. One way of constituting the boundaries of complex systems is to focus on place. Castellani et al provide a detailed definition in this respect:

> people and places need to be integrated; related, places need to be thought of in holistic or systems terms as complex, emergent entities; furthermore, places need to be seen as functioning at multiple levels of scale; operating at open-ended boundaries; fluid, mobile and evolving; not constrained by traditional notions of space and time; comprised of nonlinear feedback loops and causal pathways; with subjective histories and multiple social meanings; emerging out of the intersection between micro and macro, the local and the global, and agency and structure; and, finally, as nodes in a larger network of places and environmental forces. In short, places need to be treated as complex systems. (2012: 2)

Matheson et al assert that 'analysis of health inequalities has emphasised geographic area as it has been shown, through various measures of socio-economic position, that there is an enduring relationship between geography and health outcomes' (2009: 221). Curtis (2008) identifies how the European Union, member countries and more local administrations all have policies and projects that aim to influence the economic or social conditions for the population, or to modify the physical environment. She notes that 'these have the potential to change the social, economic and physical determinants of health and to produce short or long-term changes in public health' (2008: 293).

Much of the discussion about complexity theory so far has been relatively abstract, which supports Greenhalgh's assertion that complexity theory, 'is little more than a general world view at a high level of abstraction; it needs to be refined adapted and applied in different ways for different research questions' (2009: 1). Given the focus of this book, Klijn and Snellen's (2009) application of complexity theory to public administration is particularly useful here. They concentrate on three dimensions of complexity theory – non-linear dynamics, self-organisation and co-evolution – that are helpful in getting a handle on the complexity of policy making. We expand on these below by drawing on additional literature and applying them to the complexity of health inequalities policy making in England.

Non-linear dynamics in complexity theory

While MacIntosh et al (2006) emphasise that there are many different strands of complexity theory, a common theme is that they each attempt to understand change and the dynamics of systems as a result of the complex interaction of the parts of those systems. Klijn and Snellen (2009) identify complexity theory's focus on both linear and non-linear connections between actors and within and between complex systems as a key feature distinguishing complexity from other social science theories. Linear dynamics are where a proportional change follows an increase or repetition of incentives; non-linear dynamics are where incentives or factors can create a disproportional effect or where unexpected effects occur. Indeed, Klijn argues that, despite difference in approaches to complexity theory, a common idea is 'that the whole (the system) is greater than the sum of the parts (the individual agents), while, at the same time, developments of the whole stem from the (interaction of the) parts' (2008: 301). This complexity of non-linear dynamics can be illustrated through literature about neighbourhood decline in post-industrial societies and 'advanced marginality' (see, for example, Wilson, 1987; Wacquant, 2008). Wallace and Wallace identify the potential for relatively small perturbations of public policy or socioeconomic structure to be amplified in 'stressed human ecosystems' so that they can literally 'shatter' community structures (1997: 798). For example, Lupton and Power (2002) highlight the process of 'residential sorting', whereby the introduction of a few antisocial families can lead to more well-off families leaving the neighbourhood, which becomes increasingly undesirable and associated with social problems. These are examples of disproportional change and non-linear dynamics against the backdrop of industrial decline and post-industrial renewal. They are highly relevant to understanding the role of social determinants in the extent and structuring of health inequalities. This dynamic can also help to explain why people adopt unhealthy behaviours (see, for example, Marmot, 2010), as well as helping us to understand variations in the way people respond to advice, guidance and interventions from the state. Consequently, we must consider the influence of whether those that are most marginalised[11] appear to have less 'stake' in society and, therefore, less trust, interest and incentive in following advice about changing behaviours and accessing services.

The following two examples further illustrate the complex causal relationships associated first with a specific health condition and second with health inequalities more generally. Byrne (2011) deploys an often-used example of tuberculosis (TB), which we return to in Chapter Four, to illustrate an understanding of complex causality. The exposure of an individual human to the TB bacillus has causal potential, but whether or not that individual develops the clinical disease depends on their own genetic makeup and their general health. Byrne concludes that 'general health in turn will be a function of the whole set of circumstances they have experienced throughout their life up to the point of exposure' (2011: 22). This process of linking individual health to social determinants helps to provide explanations for variations in health status within, and between, social groups. A second example of complex causal pathways is provided by Dahlgren and Whitehead's well-known representation of 'the main determinants of health' (1991). Their model highlights the interrelated and complex relationships that influence population health by identifying a range of determinants, including general socioeconomic, economic and cultural conditions; social and community networks; individual lifestyle factors; and age, sex and constitutional factors. This model is useful for identifying a wide range of influences at different levels that are relevant to understandings of the complex health system. We would argue that alongside this mapping of individual components of such a system is a need to understand the connections between these different elements as non-linear and dynamic relationships, which potentially provide different pathways to the health outcomes experienced by individuals and populations.

Such dynamics are reinforced by fragmentation and diversity within governance systems tasked with developing local policy and action to tackle health inequalities. Indeed, further non–linear dynamics exist within these systems through the dependence of governmental organisations on a wide variety of societal organisations for the formation and implementation of policy and the delivery of public services, and through the interconnections that are linked to networks of actors and the complexity of their interactions (Klijn and Snellen, 2009). The provision of health and social care services in many advanced capitalist countries is increasingly based on a mixed economy of care, involving a growing diversity of public, private, voluntary and community providers (see, for example, Knapp et al, 2001; Peckham and Exworthy, 2003; Milligan, 2009). The plurality of commissioners and providers of services creates dynamics in health and social care systems that resonate strongly with strands of complexity. For example, Gerrits (2008) and Haynes (2008) claim that complex adaptive systems become dynamic through the ongoing actions and responses of agents. In health and social care systems, agents include (but are not limited to) service users; carers (both formal and informal); public, private, and voluntary service providers; advocacy groups; and commissioners and managers of services. These also operate across a range of scales from local government to the neighbourhood level.

Self-organisation

Klijn (2008) asserts that by understanding how systems operate at and between different levels we can generate insights into how complex integrated service delivery can be governed. Klijn and Snellen note that a particular feature of theories about complex systems is that 'many theories on complex systems stress that systems are governed by a spontaneous order: i.e. that they are self-organising' (2009: 27). They suggest that such systems have a degree of self-containment and closure and adapt to their environment but do so with properties and characteristics that are created and sustained in the system itself. As a result self-organising systems are difficult to govern and/or influence (2009: 29).

Buijs et al (2009) argue that in self-organisation there is not a central decision maker; rather, decision making is fragmented as decisions are made by several actors, possibly at several locations in space and time. Nevertheless, in setting targets and other goals, policy makers seek to manage system outcomes, not least in the context of health inequalities through requiring more or less formal partnership structures. According to Hunter et al, 'the complexities in addressing health inequalities and in improving the health of the population are reflected in a wide range of regional and local partnerships which span health services, local authorities, business and, the third sector' (2007: 2). As this wide range of actors indicates, systems dealing with health inequalities are likely to be characterised by a broad range of different – and sometimes competing – goals, with the result that not all actors accord the same degree of priority to the reduction of these inequalities. For example, commissioners may want to prioritise the reduction of health inequalities through shifting the balance of spending to prevention. However, many of the most powerful existing providers (especially acute trusts) have a predictable interest in maintaining existing patterns of resource allocation and act as significant counterweights in the production of outcomes through self-organising health systems. At the same time, objectives to reduce health inequalities do not operate in a vacuum but themselves compete for priority with the other goals of individual actors. Hence the concern to ensure that public health resources currently being transferred to local authorities are ring-fenced and cannot be diverted to other areas of local authority. A further source of complexity in systems generating inequalities of health outcomes is the extent of variations in health-seeking and health-promoting behaviours on the part of individuals and social groups. This poses challenges to service delivery and the capacity for the state to respond to the self-organisation of individuals. Indeed, Buck and Frosini (2012) note that the government needs to be smarter at working out how to engage with the very poorest; better at understanding why they drink, smoke and eat fatty food; and more perceptive about what might persuade them to change their lifestyles.

Gerrits (2008) identifies these types of systems as networks of interactions between agents, but highlights that not all the connections extend to all agents and that these connections may be temporal rather than constant. Consequently, agents in the system may or may not have complete knowledge of the system as a whole but do have agency and reflexive capacity. Indeed, the self-organising tendency of these agents is an important characteristic of these systems. Finally, it is important to recognise that the notion of self-organisation does not preclude the existence of hierarchy (Cilliers, 2001). Although the outcomes of self-organising systems are, by definition, not determined by hierarchical relationships between different structures and agents, this is not to say that hierarchy is without influence. In fact, the nature and strength of hierarchy within individual system components can be an important influence on self-organising systems. This observation is of particular significance in the field of health inequalities, where one of the two major interests (the NHS) operates through a more or less unified bureaucratic hierarchy and the other (local government) is at the centre of a set of discontinuous accountability relationships, which are downwards to local residents, outwards to local partners and upwards to central government.

Co-evolution: The mutual influence of systems on one another

According to Klijn and Snellen the concept of co-evolution relates to the idea that 'complex systems are not only complex in and of themselves but also because they are connected to other complex systems that influence one another' (2009: 29). As a result, they highlight that 'many cases in complex policy processes where strategic choices by sets of actors in one system or network are influenced, sometimes quite unexpectedly, by sets of strategic choices by other actors' (2009: 30). Consequently, the idea of connectivity applies not just to elements within a system but also to the relationship between systems (2009: 30). From this perspective, the significance of identifying many different types of social determinants of health is that each tends to exist within its individual policy system (such as employment, housing, education or welfare), in which decisions are not necessarily driven by their implications for health inequalities, but the outcomes of which may have significant consequences for their distribution and intensity. Indeed, the establishment of the NHS separate from local government institutionalised the division between personal medicine on one hand and many of the systems related to the wider determinants of health on the other. We discuss the significance of this development in more detail in Part Two of this book. However, to give an indication of co-evolution between these systems we now briefly turn to budget allocations under the 2010 Coalition government.

The Coalition Agreement (Cabinet Office, 2010a) included a commitment to increase NHS spending in real terms. As a result, the NHS was exempted from the intended reduction in public spending overall. In consequence, local government was required to take a disproportionate share of spending cuts (amounting to 26% of its budget in real terms over four years, according to the Public Accounts Committee (2013)). Since adult social care constitutes the largest single budget head in local authorities, it was inevitable that its spending share would be seriously threatened. With the cost–effective use of NHS resources closely dependent upon the provision of social care, we see the mutual influence of policy choices about one system on another. For example, the Public Accounts Committee (2013) expressed concerns about the lack of understanding of the effects of funding changes on local authorities for other services, such as whether there will be increases in hospital costs as patients wait longer to be discharged and emergency readmissions go up.

A further example of co-evolution is provided by Kelly's call for a relational understanding of 'changing, overlapping and coalescing groups and the ways these influence vulnerability, exposure, risk and health' (2010: 268). He argues that social class or socioeconomic grouping and ethnicity and gender are relational, and that at the heart of these relationships are fundamental conflicts over power, access to resources and life chances more generally. In this respect, Gerrits' characterisation of co-evolution as 'the result of various patterns that drive the mutual adjustment of systems and agents within systems' (2008: 5) becomes highly relevant. To this we must add the broader influence of the macroeconomic environment described earlier in this chapter, which also co-evolves with these sets of social circumstances.

Conclusion

In this chapter we have sought to develop our understanding of health inequalities in relation to: the socially structured nature of health and how recognising the interactions between individual and social levels of health are essential in shaping interventions to improve health; different political and ideological conceptions of inequality and how these influence both the social determinants of health and the policy responses to these; and wicked problems and the need to select methodological approaches capable of dealing with these. Developing our understanding in this way has led us to complexity-based approaches that seek to avoid reductionism in isolating human agency and structures, and instead to concentrate on the interactions between these. However, much health research (including MRC and some National Institute for Health Research guidance) is based on a fundamentally different approach to understanding social reality, namely the hierarchy of evidence privileging experimental research design.

Why does this matter? Let's take the example of self-organisation and how this might relate to the implementation of policies to tackle health inequalities. The discussion about self-organisation in the chapter mainly focuses on the implications of different administrative responses to health inequalities. However, the Ron Swanson quote towards the start of the chapter draws attention to different ideological conceptions and how they may influence individuals' responses to the state, while the section on non-linear dynamics highlights how unequal stakeholding in society may marginalise groups and individuals. Both of these positions lead to suspicion about the role of the state and its interventions, but as consequences of quite different types of self-organisation – those grounded in libertarianism and those grounded in advanced marginality. It follows that public policy on health inequalities (in particular, in relation to incentivising people to adopt healthier behaviours) has to address both the neoliberal hostility to an interventionist or 'nanny state' and also the marginalisation of groups, which many would regard as a by-product of the neoliberal project. Consequently, understanding such dynamics is important for both research and practice in the field of health inequalities and is likely to involve reconciling this self-organisation with the histories and contexts in which these individuals are embedded. In so doing, the temptation to control, isolate and reduce components of dynamic and integrated systems to discrete elements must be resisted, as this abstracts the problem of health inequalities in terms of how individuals' motivations and behaviours are shaped. The next chapter provides an example of a whole system approach to conceptualising health inequalities across English local authority areas with high levels of deprivation. This approach encourages researchers, policy makers and practitioners to consider the roles of context and agency and the interactions between these.

THREE

Health inequalities: adopting a whole system approach

Introduction

It has been argued in the preceding chapters that health inequalities are complex and require policy and research approaches that account for this. Developing whole system approaches can be an important step in responding to this complexity. This approach is closely aligned with Lazarsfeld's (1937) notion of 'property spaces', which defines 'attributes' that are considered relevant to the outcomes (in our case health inequalities) under investigation. Ragin (2000) extends Lazarsfeld's and Barton's (1955) property space approach to study cases as configurations. This chapter reflects on research that applies Ragin's qualitative comparative analysis (QCA) methodology to identify key features of health and social care systems in terms of local policy and practice, ways of working, types of interventions and local contextual conditions. The main focus of this chapter is on the conditions[12] that comprise a whole system approach to understanding health inequalities. Prior to this the development of area-based approaches to tackling health inequalities and the importance of local context are considered. The chapter concludes with a section on the binary nature of causation and how this can be related to complexity.

Area-based approaches to tackling health inequalities

England's neighbourhood renewal strategy (NRS) was launched in 2001 with the ambition that 'within 10 to 20 years no-one should be seriously disadvantaged by where they live' (Social Exclusion Unit, 2001). Six years later the programme was wound up, regarded as having failed to deliver much measurable change in the 88 deprived local authority areas targeted with some £3 billion of additional spending (Barber, 2008; AMION Consulting, 2010). In its place came a much more focused programme, the Working Neighbourhoods Fund, resourcing local interventions to tackle worklessness.

The author's (Blackman) own experience of the NRS was both as an academic working in urban policy and public health and as a practitioner. This latter role came about from being recruited as a 'neighbourhood renewal adviser' by the central government department running the strategy – initially the Office of the Deputy Prime Minister and later the Department for Communities and Local Government (DCLG). Neighbourhood renewal advisers worked as consultants to local partnerships responsible for delivering the NRS in their areas, and the main job was to advise on how to improve health outcomes. The abandonment and apparent failure of the NRS is therefore a personal as well as a public story. The experience was a rich source of ideas and material for a book, *Placing health: Neighbourhood renewal, health improvement and complexity* (Blackman, 2006), inspired not primarily by engagement with scholarship but by engagement with practice. However, a central argument of this chapter is that although this policy programme was ended prematurely it made an important contribution to my scholarship in helping to frame health inequality not as a problem of relationships between variables but as a problem to do with the states of whole systems.

One reading of the short history of the NRS is that it was just another instance of area-based initiatives failing because the underlying causes of inequality lie beyond local geography in the social relations of capitalism itself (Pantazis and Gordon, 2000; Ball and Maginn, 2004). An alternative reading, and one favoured by the UK's New Labour government elected in 1997, was that such initiatives failed because they were not rigorously performance managed to deliver their outcomes. The NRS, therefore, was replete with targets for narrowing the gap across worklessness, crime, education achievement, health, housing conditions, the physical environment and liveability. This reflected the embrace of 'command–and–control' performance management that characterised New Labour's approach to intervention, but it also marked 'a much firmer statement of the desirability of a more spatially equal society than governments have ever voiced before' (Kintrea and Morgan, 2005: 13). One consequence was that success or failure would be more public and explicit than previously in programmes of this type.

Running in parallel with the NRS was a national strategy to tackle health inequality in England, which had a strong area-based element focused on a 'Spearhead' group of 70 local authority areas with the highest rates of deprivation and mortality (DH, 2003; 2004a). These areas largely overlapped with the NRS areas. The health inequality strategy continued until Labour was defeated in the 2010 general election and replaced with a Coalition government of Conservatives and Liberal Democrats. The strategy was also characteristically shaped by a command-and-control approach to targets for narrowing gaps between local measures and national averages by the year 2010, principally in life expectancy. The new Coalition government's hostility to national targets performance managed from the centre meant that the strategy was abandoned, although it too appeared to have failed.

Although the NRS recorded some modest changes for the better, especially in worklessness and education, health inequality measured in terms of life expectancy gaps continued to widen during the period of both these strategies (AMION Consulting, 2010). Mackenbach (2011) claimed that the strategy failed because of too much emphasis on downstream interventions and too little on upstream interventions, and insufficient scale. However, this judgement may be premature according to Bambra's (2012) analysis of recent data on infant mortality, which shows a narrowing class gap. Both authors, though, ignore some apparent notable achievements of the strategy regarding two of its underpinning targets for reducing premature mortality from cancers and circulatory disease. These mortality rates fell sharply across the country, but even more sharply in deprived areas, narrowing the gap for two major causes of death (DH, 2009). Why these gaps should narrow while life expectancy gaps widen is a complex issue. For example, falling mortality from cancers and heart disease will partly reflect improving survival rates following treatment – and coincide with rising morbidity – while life expectancy will reflect deeper and longer-term processes such as the health damage caused by working in heavy industry and long-term unemployment, both of which are typical of many deprived areas and have a long reach over the lifespan (Blackman, 2006).

In fact, cancers and circulatory disease targets are more valid than life expectancy for programmes like the health inequality and neighbourhood renewal strategies because they can be related more easily to theories of change based on feasible interventions. This is reflected in the work to model interventions necessary to achieve mortality reductions in the Spearhead areas undertaken by the London Health Observatory (Association of Public Health Observatories, 2007). Their modelling used smoking quit rates and hypertensive and statin treatment rates. This clear bias towards downstream rather than upstream interventions was justified on the grounds that these types of intervention had a better evidence base to enable this kind of modelling than evidence about wider determinants, and were likely to have a quicker effect (Blackman, 2006). The fact that the inputs to and outputs from these models were numbers no doubt added to their attractiveness to policy makers, with quantification giving an apparently 'scientific' status to the work.

Chapter Eight reflects on the results of a study that adopted a rather different approach to modelling 'what works' in tackling health inequalities, applying the approach of using logical reasoning based on case membership of sets called QCA. This research used conditions – selected by the researchers along with public health practitioners – that were thought to be important to narrowing mortality gaps and teenage conception rates in the Spearhead areas. A first stage of co-production focused on the development of a data collection instrument with expert stakeholders to enable the search for complex and multiple causes in relation to programme outcomes through deploying systematic cross-case comparisons. The objective was to find out what works when, and where, with the explicit recognition that multiple complex causal configurations can be related to outcome conditions. A co-interpretation phase of the project involved meetings held with sets of expert stakeholders where results were presented for collective discussion. These also served a purpose in disseminating examples of effective practice in relation to the achievement of objectives. This direct route to impact was reinforced by a final report that was prepared and circulated to all participating primary care trusts (PCTs), which included the overall results of the study and an individual profile of their area. These provided 'bespoke' comparisons of local working practices, contextual characteristics and outcomes, enabling those PCTs not narrowing their health inequalities to identify missing conditions that might enable them to narrow their gaps. We invited PCTs to contact us for further information or advice, and several requests for more detailed reports and meetings were met. The report also attracted the attention of the Audit Commission and the National Audit Office (NAO). A meeting was held with the former to discuss the results, and the author was invited to join the NAO's Expert Panel for its investigation into tackling inequalities in life expectancy, published in July 2010 (NAO, 2010).

The importance of context

The London Health Observatory models were classic reductionist medical statistics, using associations between variables to infer outcomes for individuals. Kelly (2010) argues how this kind of 'variable-based' technique averages across many individuals, not accounting for determinants that operate at levels above and beyond individuals. Of just as much concern is their use of evidence from randomised controlled trials (RCTs), where the external validity of the RCTs is unknown (Cartwright, 2007a). The large emphasis put on treatment with statins and anti-hypertensives in the later stages of the neighbourhood renewal and health inequality strategies was not based on evidence about actual effectiveness because this evidence, from actual implementation in real world settings, was not available (Järvinen et al, 2011). Dispensing medication on a very large scale to people living in deprived areas, however, had plausibility for policy makers wanting to stop people dying prematurely, as did the 'hard' statistics that seemed to justify it (rightly or wrongly). There was none of the complexity of trying to get people coping with multiple disadvantages to eat more healthily, take more exercise or stop smoking, or – more fundamentally – to unravel how to prevent the injuries of manual and routine social class backgrounds.

Paradoxically, as Chapter Eight shows later, the answer to tackling this complexity is to simplify it, but not by using reductionism. Chapman explains:

> The essential aspect of the reductionist approach is that complexity is simplified by dividing a problem into sub-problems or lesser components ... The operation of the original complex entity is then reconstructed from the operation of the components. But herein lies a problem. What if essential features of the entity are embedded not in the components but in their interconnectedness? What if its complexity arises from the ways in which its components actually relate to and interact with one another? ... Systems thinking has an alternative strategy for simplifying complexity, namely going up a level of abstraction. (2004: 35)

What both the neighbourhood renewal and health inequality strategies did was to frame their targeted local authority areas as systems. While it might be argued just how real a system a local government area is, it is a reasonable representation of Meadows' definition that 'a system is an interconnected set of elements that is coherently organized in a way that achieves something', to which she added that all systems have elements, interconnections and a function or purpose (2009: 11). Indeed, the targeted areas all had something called local strategic partnerships (LSPs) – forums tasked with achieving just these characteristics of interconnection, coherent organisation and purpose across local services and in relation to the neighbourhood renewal and health inequality targets.

Nutley et al conceptualise this level of policy system as 'the meso or organisational policy level' (2007: 77), a relatively neglected contextual level in the policy literature, at which factors such as organisational culture come into play. Although overlooked in the literature, however, this level was given a priority in policy making by the neighbourhood renewal and health inequality strategies. This was not about some naïve view that the solutions to inequality lay at a local level of intervention, but rather based on an understanding that national economic and social policies would not be enough to turn around local areas with concentrated problems.

The spatial sorting of markets filters people into areas of more or less relative affluence, but the areas themselves bring to this mix important attributes such as the quality and safety of the physical environment and how well services are run. The clustering of these compositional and contextual conditions creates uneven geographies of outcome, including health outcomes. Just as importantly, it creates an uneven landscape for any policy intervention to interact with, shaping not just how – and whether – the intervention 'works' but also the nature of the intervention itself, such as different emphases across its elements and different qualities of local leadership and relationships.

The strong performance management of the neighbourhood renewal and health inequality strategies reflected a view in government that past urban programmes had been heavy on strategy but light on delivery (Atkinson et al, 2006). 'Low-performing' local authorities were seen to be part of this problem; the Commission on Social Justice, set up by an earlier Labour government, argued against channelling programmes though local authorities (Commission on Social Justice, 1994). The NRS was to be delivered by LSPs, accountable to regional offices of central government. Local authorities would be one of several local organisations represented on the LSP, which included the PCT responsible for commissioning local health services. The NRS made all these organisations accountable for local delivery of national 'floor targets'. These were innovative inequality targets based on narrowing gaps between local measures and national averages. They spanned education, employment, enterprise, crime, housing, liveability, health, road accidents and regional economic growth. Three of the health floor targets were to narrow these gaps in teenage pregnancies and premature mortality from cancers and circulatory diseases. An important part of the role of neighbourhood renewal advisers was to work with LSPs on floor target action plans that aligned activities with the targets in a theory of change model. This was a significant challenge, since what was being aimed at was making faster progress in the targeted areas than the national rates of improvement, and thus narrowing the gap.

In December 2005, the author received an assignment from the Government Office for the North West (GONW) asking him to investigate the reasons behind a variable level of achievement across the 21 neighbourhood renewal areas in north-west England. Six of the LSPs had a narrowing gap in circulatory disease mortality, 11 had a narrowing gap in cancers mortality and 10 had a narrowing gap in teenage conceptions. Most of the LSPs had experienced widening gaps since the inception of the NRS, but the picture was not consistent. All three gaps were narrowing in only one LSP, and similarly there was only one LSP where all three gaps were widening.

The conventional approach to this kind of scenario is to carry out some interviews in the areas with narrowing gaps and seek to identify good practice for wider dissemination. The problem with this approach is causal attribution when there are not systematic like-with-like comparisons across areas with both narrowing and widening gaps. In discussing this with Dave Byrne, he suggested using QCA. The assignment became a QCA study and was published in 2010 (Blackman and Dunstan, 2010).

While variable-based methods such as regression estimate the average effects of independent variables, which may or often may not be reflected in individual cases, QCA is a method for explaining why specific cases have particular outcomes, with an outcome analysed as the product of how conditions combine together to produce it (Ragin, 2000). Chapter Eight discusses this in more detail; in this chapter the discussion is confined to the importance of conditions in this whole system approach to causal modelling.

Conditions in whole systems

What conditions could be important in determining whether some areas in north-west England have narrowing health inequalities while others have widening gaps? Each neighbourhood renewal area is a case, but also a local system with organisational attributes and contextual features applying across each system and representing its conditions. The outcome condition, narrowing or widening over a defined period of time, was a given (although requiring judgements about measurement not considered here). The causal conditions were a question needing theoretical and substantive knowledge, both tacit and codified. For example, in tackling health inequalities locally, services may be reactive or proactive; interactions between agents may be more or less aligned to common goals; and contextual conditions such as organisational leadership, aspirations and demographic, ethnic and socioeconomic factors may have a wide range of states that have effects on outcomes.

In the GONW study, the conditions were derived by searching the literature and engaging practitioners in workshops, from which longlists of conditions thought likely to affect the outcomes were derived. Some of the data for these conditions was available from secondary sources: the Index of Multiple Deprivation; a liveability index (Collinge et al, 2005); proportions of the total local population aged16–19 years, aged 65 years and over, and in minority ethnic groups; and people who moved address in the previous year (all 2001 census). However, much had to be collected from the LSPs as primary data, using specially designed self-assessment questionnaires completed by small teams in each of the areas, principally addressing local ways of working and types of intervention. All conditions were eventually operationalised as variables and explored using the statistical package for the social sciences (SPSS) for patterns of relationships with the outcomes. Shortlists of conditions were then identified and used in the QCA models.

Academic research aims to produce the best possible knowledge, but an important test for policy research is that the results prove useful because they enable practitioners to make evidence-based decisions. The following sections consider why binarised conditions based on a quality being either present or absent are useful for decision making where the decisions are also binary: to do (a) or (b). But for now it is noted that the results for GONW were received with a lot of interest, extensively discussed and widely disseminated as evidence supporting what needed to be done where the gap was not narrowing.

Subsequently, the author worked with Dave Byrne on a successful proposal to the National Institute for Health Research to carry out a QCA study across all of England's Spearhead areas to understand what was behind some areas narrowing their gaps and others not. Jonathan Wistow was hired as a researcher on the project, and the resources available meant that both the scale and depth of the research were improvements on the GONW study, particularly the time to draw together much more extensive secondary data and to develop the questionnaires in consultation with a range of stakeholders. The questionnaires, for example, incorporated recent developments in policy and practice, especially in commissioning practice, and extensive advice from the national Health Inequalities Support Team, who were engaged in a series of visits to Spearhead areas. The downside of this was that the questionnaires evolved significantly from the GONW study, making it difficult to compare results, although some like–with–like comparisons were possible.[13] The GONW questionnaires were the starting point for designing the new versions but were revised following a detailed review of literature on tackling health inequalities. A mini-Delphi process was then used with three groups of expert stakeholders: the Department of Health (DH)'s national support teams for health inequalities and teenage pregnancies, and three regional workshops with local practitioners from Spearhead areas, representing a variety of role types. With the national support teams this took the form of developing the questionnaires through a series of drafting iterations, sharing the reasoning for each set of changes until final drafts were agreed. With the workshops that followed, it took the form of a structured discussion about content, design and phrasing, finalising these by consolidating agreement around preferred options.

The research involved innovation both in data construction and in data analysis. These were not entirely separate processes, in that we constructed our data and undertook the analyses in dialogue with informed stakeholders, both in workshops and dedicated meetings. Effective policy – its design, implementation and evaluation – depends on several evidentiary bases. These are all involved directly or indirectly in the development and assessment of 'good programmes' and help us to understand effectiveness in a more practical and contextual way.

Our approach was to see what different data sources might tell us and we did this through the three lenses described by Head (2007): scientific research-based knowledge, which derives from systematic analysis of conditions, trends and interrelationships; practical implementation knowledge, which is a combination of the day-to-day experiential knowledge of practitioners and the management, or organisational knowledge of those involved in policy and programme implementation; and political knowledge, which is the sum of the knowledge held in all its forms by political actors. We did not access political knowledge for the data-gathering phase of the study since our focus was on local strategic and management actors, but we considered its influence in interpreting some of our findings. For example, the results on bureaucratic practices reported in Chapter Eight are considered through the political lens and the influence of 'audit culture' on local practice. The emphasis at the time of our research on measures that could have a short-term effect on health inequalities reflected the political imperative behind meeting 2010 targets (Blackman et al, 2009).

Questionnaire design

The questionnaires were divided into two sections. They are described here in some detail because they represent our synthesis of what is known about what works in tackling health inequalities locally, which we define as conditions in local whole systems. Interestingly, when we came to analyse the effects of these conditions, few mattered to the outcomes, and those that did mattered in combination with others.

The first section of the questionnaires focused on policy and practice. Respondents were asked to self-assess against descriptions of achievement on a six-point scale from 'less than basic' to 'exemplary' and to provide examples to back up their assessments. Confidentiality and anonymity of particular areas were assured under a National Health Service (NHS)-approved ethics protocol. The questions covered the following eight topics, each described briefly and identifying how initial drafts were informed by the literature but amended with practitioner input from the mini–Delphi consultations in a process of co–production.

1. Identifying, understanding and targeting the inequalities gap in the Spearhead area (all questionnaires). An effective process for identifying, understanding and targeting health inequalities would seem to be an important first step in tackling them (Hunter and Killoran, 2004; DH, 2007b). A question was designed with descriptions of basic to exemplary practice and considered in the first round of mini–Delphi consultations. It was agreed that the question should be included, subject to revision. Taking the example of the cancers questionnaire, the following phrasing was suggested initially for the descriptor of 'basic' practice and was unamended following the mini–Delphi process:

> Recent and trend data on cancer incidence, the pattern of cancers, mortality and survival rates are readily available and used to identify priorities and plan interventions aimed at narrowing the area's cancers gap.

'Good' practice was initially described as:

> All of 'basic' plus data about premature mortality are complemented by local data on disease prevalence, risk factors, lifestyles and accessibility of services from QOF [the Quality and Outcomes Framework],[14] surveys or other local studies. Data are as up-to-date as possible and trends are analysed. National targets are translated into local targets with planned trajectories for meeting them. Data

are monitored to track progress over time towards meeting targets to 2010 and beyond. This monitoring is used to plan and review services, with resulting changes to policies and service specifications where more impact is needed to meet targets. Efforts are made to collect data by social class and ethnic group.

Following the mini–Delphi process this descriptor was amended, mainly to place more emphasis on 'joined-up' practice, and became:

All of 'basic' plus cancer data are analysed and compared at district and small area/practice levels. Recent and trend data are available on risk factors associated with the cancers contributing most to the cancers gap (from surveys and/or QOF). Efforts are made to collect and analyse data by social class, ethnic group, gender and other indicators of inequality and diversity. There is a clear relationship between data analysis and types and scales of intervention, including how cancer contributes to the Spearhead area's life expectancy gap. There are reporting mechanisms that identify progress against milestones to meet targets. Reporting mechanisms of different systems/ partners are compatible.

The 'exemplary' descriptor was initially drafted as:

All of 'good' plus this is leading to demonstrable changes in the way services are delivered, with evidence from evaluations that this is driving progress against health inequality targets. Data are available for small neighbourhoods and target groups. Service providers are trained and skilled in understanding how what they do can widen or narrow health inequalities and are using this knowledge to change the way they deliver services.

This was revised following the mini–Delphi consultations to place more emphasis on some specifics of evidence-based practice and targeting, and became:

All of 'good' plus the cancers gap, its causes and its contribution to the life expectancy gap are sufficiently understood to know what interventions are needed, where and on what scale. These interventions are implemented, monitored and reviewed, considering where more impact is needed to narrow the gap. Problems of late presentation and low screening uptake are investigated and initiatives targeted on hard to reach groups. Service providers are trained and skilled in understanding how and what they do can either widen or narrow inequalities, and are using this knowledge to change the way they deliver services. Data analysis leads to demonstrable changes in service delivery.

2. The role of commissioning (all questionnaires). A question about commissioning was not included in the initial draft questionnaires but was added following the mini-Delphi process. This was done to take into account the evolution of policy to promote improved commissioning of health services by local PCTs, especially the introduction of the so-called 'world class commissioning' initiative (DH, 2007c). Commissioning involves assessing the health needs of patients and populations, and ensuring that services are available to meet them.

Taking the cardiovascular disease (CVD) questionnaire as our example, the initial phrasing of the 'basic' practice descriptor was amended during the process to include: 'Services accommodate national referral-to-treatment targets and the impact of new targets on capacity is accommodated in developmental plans.' The following addition was made to the 'exemplary' descriptor: 'There are joint plans, planning processes, contracts, management and information systems across all relevant stakeholders. Service standards are explicitly detailed in SLAs [service level agreements].' Some changes to phrasing were also made to remove ambiguity and align better with practice vocabularies.

3. Partnership working across sectors at a strategic level in the Spearhead area (all questionnaires). The significance of strategic partnership working in reducing health inequalities is identified by the DH (2007c), Exworthy and Powell (2004) and Hunter et al (2007), among others. A question was designed with descriptions of basic to exemplary practice and taken through the mini-Delphi process. Taking the example of the teenage conceptions questionnaire, the initial 'basic' descriptor was amended to include: 'Progress reports are received from a Teenage Pregnancy Partnership Board/equivalent body with senior PCT, Children's Services, Youth Services and third sector representation.' The 'good' descriptor was amended to include: 'A coordinator ensures actions are carried out. There is a coordinated approach to identifying those at risk.' The 'exemplary' descriptor was amended to include: 'Trusting relationships between the key agencies lead to shared resources and joint planning/contracting across health services, children's services and worklessness.'

4. Local services working together on the ground in the Spearhead area (all questionnaires). Partnership working between frontline services would seem to be another important factor in tackling health inequalities (Sassi, 2005; Brigden, 2006; Hunter et al, 2007). Using the example of the cancers questionnaire, the first draft 'basic' practice descriptor was amended to include: 'Frontline relationships work well between primary and secondary care and local authority staff, with established cross-referral practices and a common agenda prioritising greatest needs.' The following addition was made to the 'exemplary' descriptor: 'Residents and users are often involved with frontline staff in decision-making, with special measures to reach and raise aspirations for better services among the most disadvantaged.'

5. Community engagement in the Spearhead area (cancers and CVD questionnaires). A question about community engagement was included to explore the impact that this might be having on health outcomes and to respond to the growing significance of community engagement in both the academic and policy literature. For example, the DH (2007c: 17) identifies empowering disadvantaged communities to aspire to good health as a high impact change for both the NHS and local government to narrow health inequalities. Brigden (2006), Cropper (2002) and Hunter and Killoran (2004) suggest that community engagement can play an important role in narrowing health inequality gaps. Consequently, a question was designed with descriptions of basic to exemplary practice. Taking the example of the CVD questionnaire, the 'basic' practice descriptor was amended to include: 'One-off consultation (such as a workshop) is more common than longer-term community engagement.' The 'exemplary' descriptor was amended to include: 'There are demonstrable impacts on health-seeking behaviours likely to narrow the CVD gap. Mechanisms are in place to evaluate and learn from community engagement.'

6. The public health workforce in this Spearhead area (or the children and young people's workforce for the teenage conceptions questionnaire). This question was not in the first draft of the questionnaire but was included following a suggestion made during the mini-Delphi process. Public health workforce planning and capacity have been identified as important in narrowing health inequalities (Berridge, 2007; DH, 2007b; Fotaki, 2007; Hunter et al, 2007). Fotaki (2007) writes that adequate skills and capacity are prerequisites for PCTs to focus proactively on reducing inequalities. A question was designed with descriptions of basic to exemplary practice.

Using the example of the cancers questionnaire, the 'good' practice descriptor was amended during the mini–Delphi process to include: 'There is clear leadership of public health workforce planning.' The 'exemplary' descriptor was amended to include: 'There are long term plans to develop the right skills mix and capacity for prevention and engagement.'

7. Contraception and sexual health services in the local authority area (teenage conceptions questionnaire only). The importance of contraception and sexual health services in reducing teenage conception rates are highlighted in many policy and practice documents (Department for Education and Skills, 2006a; 2006b; DCLG, 2007; DH, 2007c). A question was designed with descriptions of basic to exemplary practice and taken through the mini–Delphi process. The descriptor of 'good' practice was amended to include: 'Access is convenient and prompt in a range of settings, including multi-agency drop in services, consistent quality and choice, out of hours and young people friendly.' The 'exemplary' descriptor was amended to include: 'Contraceptive and sexual health services are highly visible and meet "You're Welcome" criteria.'

8. Smoking cessation services in the Spearhead area (cancers questionnaire but also used in the CVD analysis). The DH (2007c) and NICE (2008) highlight the importance of smoking cessation for narrowing health inequality. A question was designed with descriptions of basic to exemplary practice. The following amendment to the phrasing of the 'good' descriptor was made: 'Smoking cessation support is available in a range of community, primary and secondary care settings for everyone who smokes.' The 'exemplary' descriptor was amended to include: 'Monitoring systems ensure health professionals have access to information on the smoking status of their patients, advice offered and the response to that advice.'

These eight topics formed part 1 of the questionnaire. Part 2 contained questions focusing on ways of working, types of intervention and the local context. The questions in this section were also informed by academic and policy literature as well as practitioner and national support team input. They included the following.

- **Approaches to tackling the cancers/CVD gap or reducing teenage conception rates.** This was framed as 'a few major programmes', 'many smaller projects', or 'an integrated systematic approach' (Asthana and Halliday, 2006; DH, 2007c).

- **The frequency of progress reviews by the appropriate partnership board.** This was defined as monthly, quarterly, six-monthly, annually or not yet done (Smith, 2005).
- **Nature of the area's working culture**. Precoded options were that initiatives relied on individual commitment and champions; on a widely shared 'team player' spirit; or on good plans and systems largely independently of who is involved (Blackman and Dunstan, 2010).
- **Approach to prioritising health inequality interventions**. This question focused on whether closing the gap between the locality and the national average or reducing inequalities within the locality was the main priority, or whether these were equal priorities (Graham, 2004; DH, 2005; Walsh et al, 2007).
- **Prioritisation of the cancers/CVD gap or of reducing teenage conceptions**. This asked whether the outcome was the top priority; one of a small number of top priorities; one of a larger number of priorities; or not a priority (DH, 2005; 2007c).
- **Nature of joint meetings**. Precoded options were whether these were about funding for projects; working with shared goals and budgets; finding 'win wins'; whether there was clarity about what needed to be done and who would do it; and whether questions were asked about those not meeting targets (Exworthy and Powell, 2004; DH, 2005; 2007b).
- **Use of available evidence**. This asked about the balance between use of national evidence and guidance, and the use of local research (Graham, 2004).
- **Relative priority between primary care and reaching individuals who need early treatment on the one hand and environmental and community-wide measures on the other (cancers and CVD)**. For teenage conceptions, this question asked what was the relative priority between contraceptive and sexual health services reaching individuals at risk on the one hand and intervening in the wider determinants at a community level on the other (DH, 2000a; 2000b; 2007c; Department for Education and Skills, 2006a; 2006b; DCLG, 2007).
- **Balance between intervening in community or workplace settings (cancers and CVD), and balance between intervening in community or school and college settings (teenage conceptions)** (Department for Education and Skills, 2006a; 2006b; DCLG, 2007; DH, 2007c).

- **Leadership in the Spearhead area**. Precoded options were excellent, good, fair, poor or a mixed picture (DH, 2005; Hunter et al, 2007).
- **Organisational culture**. Options were very aspirational, quite aspirational, comfortable with the current situation or complacent and inward-looking (Hunter and Killoran, 2004; Berridge, 2007; Fotaki, 2007; Hunter et al, 2007).
- **The local strategic partnership or health partnership**. Options were that it sets clear direction, is a useful forum but not especially directive, is largely passive or presents a mixed picture (DH, 2005; Hunter et al, 2007).

Examples of how the questions were developed through the mini–Delphi process are as follows.

- **Question 1: Which of the following statements best characterises the approach in this Spearhead area to tackling the cancers gap?** Asthana and Halliday (2006) and the DH (2007c) argue that the scale and extent of approaches are important to reducing health inequalities. A question was designed and taken through the process to capture this aspect. This was initially phrased as 'a few major interventions and projects' and 'many smaller initiatives', and became amended to 'a few major programmes' and 'many smaller projects'. In addition, a third category of 'an integrated systematic approach' was added.
- **Question 8: Which of the following best describes the relative priority in this Spearhead area between: (a) a focus on tackling the cancers gap using primary care and reaching individuals who need early treatment, and (b) environmental and community-wide measures such as tobacco control, improving access to healthy foods and better housing and neighbourhoods?** The importance of both primary care and community measures in tackling health inequalities is identified by the DH (2000; 2007c). Separate questions were initially developed to include in part 2 of the questionnaire but the mini–Delphi process resulted in agreement on a single question to ask about the relative balance between two approaches in the Spearhead area.

Secondary data

A wide variety of secondary data was considered alongside the questionnaire data. This included the following.

- **performance assessment ratings**: PCT rating and local authority comprehensive performance assessment (CPA) star rating and 'direction of travel';
- **Local area information**: Index of Multiple Deprivation 2007 score, concentration and extent; overall crime rate; liveability score calculated by MORI for every local authority area in England and based on a combination of resident survey responses about the visual quality of their neighbourhood and the proportion of housing stock that is terraced or high-rise (Collinge et al, 2005); local authority migration estimates for inflow and outflow; and percentage of the working age population without a level 2 qualification;[15]
- **Health services information**: accident and emergency hospital admissions for 2005/06; QOF data on the proportion of primary care practices classified as outliers on performance measures; the proportion of single handed practices in areas; and the number of GPs in areas (excluding retainers and registrars) per 100,000 population;
- **Spend**: percentage over or under PCT target budget allocation and spend per head on cancers and CVD in 2005/06;
- **Education data** (for the teenage conceptions outcome): percentage achieving level 4+ at key stage 2 (English, maths and science); percentage achieving level 5+ at key stage 3 (English, maths and science); percentage achieving 5+ GCSEs at grades A*-C including maths and English; percentage achieving any GCSE passes; half days missed in secondary schools (overall); and percentage of 16–17 year-olds participating in education and work-based learning;
- **2001 Census demographic data**: percentage of the population that are not white; percentage of the population under 18; and percentage of the population over 65.

Conditions for a QCA study

In the QCA study, further discussed in Chapter Eight, data from the questionnaires and the secondary data sources were coded for analysis using SPSS and the qualitative comparative analysis package fsQCA. The fsQCA package works out combinations of conditions associated with given outcomes: in this case, whether or not health inequalities had been narrowing over the past few years.

It will be apparent from the above account that this was an extensive longlist of conditions, but all had one reason or another to be regarded as important influences (as key attributes of health and social care systems) on whether Spearhead areas were narrowing their gaps.

The number of conditions selected by the mini–Delphi process was around 60 for each outcome, an impossibly large number of conditions for QCA because the number of possible logical combinations of conditions would far exceed the number of cases. This means that the empirically observed cases would occupy only a tiny proportion of the potential logical space of a QCA. Berg-Schlosser and De Meur (2009) identify this as the 'limited diversity' problem, when 'the observed data are far less rich than the potential property space delineated by the conditions' (2009: 27). We needed, therefore, to select a limited number of conditions because the danger is that otherwise only a *description* will be obtained, rather than establishing core elements of possible causal mechanisms leading to the outcomes.

Berg-Schlosser and De Meur (2009) set out some good practice points for the selection of conditions in small and intermediate-N research designs, as follows.

- Conditions must vary across the cases.
- The number of conditions should be kept relatively low (approximately 6–7 for 10–40 cases) so as not to individualise cases.
- A good balance between the number of cases and conditions will most often be found through trial and error.
- Formulate a clear hypothesis for each condition regarding its connection to the outcome.

What is very interesting from the analysis, as already noted and discussed further in Chapter Eight, is that few conditions turned out to be important and, where they were, their effects were in combination with other conditions. Some conditions, however, were *necessary* in configurations sufficient to produce an outcome. This illustrates the extent of challenge for policy makers, since the absence of only one necessary condition means that the outcome will not happen. There can, though, be more than one way of achieving the outcome and the combinations of conditions can be viewed as alternative pathways to outcomes.

Causation is binary even if it is complex

The author first heard the term 'causation is binary' used on the radio several years ago by the philosopher Helen Beebee. The comment suggests that a practical decision about using dichotomised conditions in QCA also had an ontological justification (although this remains fiercely debated among philosophers).

The QCA technique employed in the Spearheads study has its roots in the earliest and most widely used application of the method developed by Ragin and now known as 'crisp set' QCA. This is based on Boolean algebra, which uses binary data based on a quality being either present or absent. It relies on the dichotomisation of variables. Thus, a Spearhead case could be coded 'crisply' as having an exemplary or good understanding and targeting of health inequalities, or not having this quality. The questionnaire has a six-point scale for evaluating this condition, so binarisation involves deciding upon the threshold at which a qualitative change in the condition makes a difference to the outcome. This is difficult if the effect is gradated, but a threshold is often apparent: there is a point in the scale at which a qualitative difference occurs.

The majority of the questions in the questionnaire used scales and the remainder had categories with some yes/no answers. The secondary data were comprised of continuous or categorical conditions. All of the conditions were explored using cross-tabulations in SPSS to establish the strength of relationship with the outcome measures and the thresholds for binarisation. These conditions were then narrowed down and further examined for their configurational relationships with the outcomes.

Judgement is involved in setting thresholds, informed by inspecting strengths of association and often numerous iterations around threshold setting, since some conditions displayed more than one skew or association in the cross-tabulations, and in these instances the condition was dichotomised two or three times (depending on the number of skews) and explored alongside other conditions in QCA data tables.

Where relationships were evident, thresholds for dichotomisation were based on where a change in relationship occurred. For example, the 'narrowing' outcome for CVD mortality was clustered in the lower range of Index of Multiple Deprivation scores, which provided the basis for binarising the scores. From the questionnaire data, there was an association between less than basic practice in public health workforce planning and a narrowing gap, but there was a clearer and stronger association between good practice or better and a not narrowing gap. Both of the thresholds had the same relationship with the outcome: narrowing to less good practice, and not narrowing to better practice (one of the counter-intuitive findings discussed briefly below). Robustness checks were undertaken to determine how binarisation thresholds affected the findings, and the thresholds used were found to be robust. We found that only a relatively small number of conditions had any patterned relationships with the outcome indicators. These were imported into fsQCA to explore their effects in combination. The provisional results from this analysis were circulated to all participating PCTs and subsequently discussed with participants at a series of workshops.

Ragin's 'fuzzy set' technique is an alternative option to crisp set that involves coding each case by the varying degree to which it belongs to sets (degrees of in- and out-ness, expressed as percentages). Potentially, the fuzzy set method makes maximum use of the information available, but dichotomisation of the data reflects a fundamental characteristic of QCA in its original form. It is easier to handle dichotomous variation in processing, and it is easier to see and interpret patterns in the form of multiple configurations of causes in output tables and reductions when we are dealing with simple presence or absence rather than degree of presence. Ragin's (2000) proposal for a 'fuzzy set social science' was intended to address exactly this issue.

As well as these practical considerations about data analysis, there is a theoretical reason for preferring dichotomised conditions when dealing with complex systems. This is because incremental changes tell us little more than that the system is in a state of dynamic equilibrium, while changes in kind point to a transition from one type of system to another. In the Spearhead study, the main interest was in differentiating systems where the health gap was narrowing with systems where it was not: two different kinds of system.

Finally, there is a third reason for preferring dichotomised conditions, which is practical decision making. Practitioners generally need to know whether to do (a) or (b), not how much a change of degree in (a) causes a change of degree in (b). If understanding and targeting of health inequalities is not good enough to narrow the gap, what level of understanding and targeting needs to be achieved to do so? In Chapter Eight we see some very interesting counter-intuitive examples of practice being 'too good', in the sense that descriptions of so-called 'best practice' were associated with a worse outcome than a 'basic' level of practice, seemingly because excessive planning and monitoring gets in the way of effective action.

Most of the narrowing/not narrowing outcomes were related to 'contradictory' configurations – that is, there were cases that contradicted general patterns. The exploratory use of QCA employs such contradictory configurations as a guide to further exploration of the data, and that is precisely what we did through revisiting the dataset and in our dialogues with practitioners in the workshops. We identified a number of plausible configurations of conditions across the dichotomised data tables and produced commentaries around these. Our study was partly intended to be a tool (a 'tin-opener') for practitioners to use to consider patterns in ways of working and local contextual conditions, but in our discussions we found we could go beyond this and consider accounts of causality.

For example, one condition was found to be necessary – although not sufficient – for Spearhead areas with narrowing cancers mortality gaps: individual commitment and championing. This condition was also absent in all the configurations where the cancers gap was not narrowing. In a good example of how quantitative data can answer 'what, when and who' questions, but is less suitable for answering 'how and why' questions, this finding meant that to understand the condition we had to draw on qualitative insights from both the literature and practitioner tacit knowledge. The questionnaire asked whether respondents either agreed or disagreed with a descriptor of what best characterised the general working culture in the Spearhead area towards narrowing the cancers gap, in which 'individual commitment and championing' was a precoded option. The question served as a tin-opener and we had to revisit the literature and our practitioner workshops to understand more about it.

The role of product champions in innovation has long been reported in the business literature, but in the health context our colleague David Hunter pointed us to Stocking's (1985) study of innovation in the NHS. She found that champions often had a key role in getting new, more effective approaches to problems taken up and diffused. Many subsequent studies have identified the role of champions in developing and disseminating process improvements and best practices. Zöllner's (2002) review of national policies for reducing social inequalities in health in Europe argues for championing as necessary for overcoming obstacles to action at both national and local levels, as does Marmot's (2010) review of progress with narrowing health inequalities in England. In our workshops with practitioners, championing of early detection and treatment was said to be key, with committed clinical leaders able to ensure that services were proactive and responsive to needs, working across organisational boundaries. Such leadership was said to animate local cancer networks. In fact, the NHS Cancer Plan put these networks at the heart of a commitment to tackle cancer: it called for them to be strongly led and for resources to be targeted where most needed (NHS, 2000).

Conclusion

The neighbourhood renewal and health inequality strategies were not failures on some important measures. More interestingly, some local areas succeeded while others failed. Important learning is possible from this experience, albeit over the short period that a favourable political environment allowed the strategies to run. This chapter has argued that this learning takes the form of a 'tale of two systems': systems with narrowing gaps and systems with gaps that were not narrowing. As simple as this dichotomy is, complexity is also evident in the different paths to the same outcome that can occur, and conditions found in one configuration being absent or acting differently in other configurations. Synergistic effects appear to arise from only certain configurations and, while some conditions are necessary, many conditions appear to be irrelevant to the outcomes. We return to these issues in our analyses of the QCA study in Chapter Eight. It is important to note now that in recognising these different paths as sets of the same types of case, practitioners can make use of the results to consider strategies that best make sense for their areas. In so doing we can take account of uneven geographies of health outcomes and consider how policy interventions interact with these.

FOUR

Measuring health inequalities

Introduction

There is very extensive literature on the measurement of health inequalities, and a conventional approach to writing a chapter on this topic would be to begin with a literature review. That will not be done here. Rather, most of this chapter will consist of a discussion of how we might measure health inequalities if we start with a complex systems frame of reference and 'a focus on the case'. So we have to start, as indeed do the better examples of the existing literature, with the following two fundamental questions:

- What is health?
- What is inequality?

For both we will attempt 'complexity theory' informed answers, but to construct those answers we also have to ask:

- What are the cases for which health inequalities should be measured?

and:

- What are the populations of those cases for which we should explore differences that we can interpret as inequalities?
- Since we are dealing with systems we also have to consider how the character of those systems changes through time. We therefore have to ask both:
- What are the trajectories of our cases through time?

and:

- How does the possibility state space change for our cases through time? That is to ask do the classificatory sets into which we allocate cases themselves change through time?[16]

71

We could summarise the set of questions above by saying we have to pay attention to what we are measuring (health and inequality) and what we are measuring it for (our cases, to which we attach the measurements). The emphasis on the plurals of cases and populations is deliberate and important. Inequality can be understood simply as difference. Carr–Hill and Chalmers–Dixon (2005) make an important distinction between inequality, which we can understand simply in terms of difference, and inequity. Inequity has a normative content, whereas inequality can be understood simply as a description of difference. In practice, the term 'health inequalities' tends to incorporate a notion of inequity – of the normative assertion that the differences observed, or more generally the degree of differences observed, should not exist and something should be done about them.

When we ask 'What is health?' we can answer this conventionally, but very usefully, by returning to the classic definition coined by the World Health Organization (WHO) in 1948: 'Health is a state of complete physical, mental and social well-being and not merely the absence of disease or infirmity' (WHO, 1948). Reading through this short document (and everybody working in or in relation to health should read it), it is clear that health as defined in these terms is first a property of individual human beings, since it asserts that good health is a fundamental right of 'every human being' – that is, people in the singular – but it goes on to refer to 'the health of all *peoples*', not of all people, as being fundamental to the attainment of peace and security. So there is both a singular and a plural conception of the entities which are entitled to good health as WHO defined it.

Measurement and complexity

The WHO definition of health refers to 'a state'. That is, in systems theory terms, it defines the proper state of a system. First, the systems of interest are individual human beings who are each unique biological, psychological and social entities. So our first interest is in the health of such entities, which we can consider as an 'effect' of the complex and interactive causal processes that generate the state of a system. Note that these causal processes include both aspects of the system itself and aspects of the whole set of other social and environmental systems which intersect with the system of interest, as well as the overall condition of the system itself. That sentence is a statement founded in the complexity frame of reference. It assigns causal powers to all of the components of the system in interaction with each other, factors external to the system in interaction with each other and with the components of the system, and the holistic system in interaction with its own components, with factors external to it and with the interactions of components and external factors. That word 'interaction' matters a great deal. Conventional statistical modelling tries, rather unsuccessfully, to cope with complex causation by entering interaction terms into linear equations. What is being asserted here is that the causes of system states are complex *and* multiple – we are also asserting the reality of equifinality – so outcomes can be the product of multiple and different causal complexes.

An illustration will demonstrate. Let us take the case of tuberculosis (TB) in a patient. If somebody gets clinical TB – that is, the person is not in a state of 'complete physical, mental and social well-being' because they are 'ill' with TB – then that condition has multiple causes. The necessary *but not sufficient* cause is exposure to the TB bacillus through coming into contact with an actively infective case. But already we have introduced complexity – there must be contact with a case. The existence of the TB bacillus in nature is not in and of itself causal. Aspects of the biological system of the individual will determine whether contact results in infection – the presence of the bacillus in the body of the individual concerned to a degree which leads to a pathology. Infection does not necessarily lead to disease, since the patient's immune system may be able to overcome the infection so that no clinical disease will result. All sorts of characteristics of the patient may influence this process, including genetic makeup and general health as a consequence of diet. If the patient has been immunised through administration of a Bacillus Calmette-Guerin (BCG) shot, that will have an effect on the movement from exposure to clinical disease. Contact will depend on social conditions, in particular overcrowding in housing, as well as on the prevalence of infective cases in the social world of the individual. Prevalence will depend on the general health levels of the population, especially in terms of adequate diet, and the effectiveness of public health measures designed both for immunisation and the rapid treatment/isolation of identified infective cases. All these elements have causal powers in relation to the initiation of the clinical disease in an individual. The development of the clinical disease for that individual is then determined (by which we mean that the outcome is either death or recovery) by the whole interaction of that patient with curative services. We have not even mentioned the biological variation in the resistance of TB strains to curative treatments. It is complex.

Historically, in societies which now have undergone the health transition – that is, moved from a condition in which many deaths were the result of infectious disease during infancy, childhood and adult life to one in which the great majority survive into 'old age' – differential rates of TB incidence, prevalence and mortality were important indicators of inequality in health across social and/or geographically defined collectivities. Both of the present author's (Byrne's) parents had siblings who died from TB in young adult life. In societies on the cusp of the health transition, such as Bangladesh (see Roy, 2012), these differences remain of very considerable importance. In societies with a high prevalence of HIV positive cases, TB remains a major subsequent cause of health inequality. And TB might very well come back to hit us all if multiple/total drug-resistant strains become globally prevalent.

The first case is always the individual who is either well or ill, although we will qualify that dichotomous description of possible systems states in a moment. However, in public health we are also interested in the health of the population as a whole, as well as of defined subgroups within it. So the subgroups are also cases, and we construct a description of these aggregates on the basis of the assemblage of microdata about individuals' health. If we continue with the TB example, we look at incidence, prevalence and death rates for the disease across some social aggregate. Given that health services, including public health, are typically delivered across an administratively defined geographical area, one kind of category is spatial. We can look at rates for sets of nation states, for individual nation states, for regions within those states, for localities within those regions and for neighbourhoods within those localities. Slum clearance procedures in the UK in the 1930s almost invariable cited TB death rates – established by inspection of death certificates which include a cause and an address – for the localities being proposed for clearance, in contrast with the general rates in the area of the local authority proposing the clearance.[17] Contrast implies difference and difference is fundamental to inequality. If we see a pattern of differences we have inequality among cases, however cased (Ragin, 1992). And where there are differences we seek a cause (which may be and usually is multiple, complex and contingent rather than singular). As MacIver asserted: '... for every difference there is a cause' (1942: 27).

If we think about the possible health system states of an individual human being, then we might begin with the ancient definition – we are quick or we are dead. That is, the system is functioning biologically or it has ceased to function. The one inevitability in this world is death.[18] We all are going to die sometime. In terms of health inequalities the issue is when we die – do we have a decent and acceptable life span before 'it is our time'? The biblical three score years and ten seems not a lot in developed societies these days, when 60 is the new 40. Death before the age of 75 is often defined as premature, although other measures include directly age-standardised mortality rates, probability of survival at a given age and years of life lost. The last is particularly interesting because before the health transition the high rates of infant and child mortality and differences among these by relevant categories were a crucial source of health inequalities.[19]

However, there is more to health state than just being alive or dead. Certainly the WHO definition requires more. We can add 'in the presence or absence of a pathological condition which limits wellbeing' – TB is an excellent example because, although an infectious disease, its natural history meant that sufferers (other than those who died as did the author's aunt of 'galloping consumption') lived with it in varying states of health for a long time and some for a whole lifetime without dying of the disease. That is to say TB could be chronic illness. We can look at individual pathologies of this kind – diabetes is a prime example, at least in terms of potential impact, as are many forms of cardiovascular disease. But there is more to chronic illness than the mere presence or absence of a single condition. Primary care physicians in particular are very well aware of the patient who presents with multiple conditions – obesity, arthritis, high blood pressure and depression is a common combination – which limit – a crucial word – their lives. All lay conceptions of health as opposed to illness assert that the difference lies in ability to function in a socially *and* age-related appropriate fashion.[20] So we have to consider the system states of individual people in terms not just of the presence of single pathologies but of a combination of conditions, which might be mutually intercausal – depression as a consequence of obesity and obesity as a recursive consequence of depression – and limiting to life. So inequalities can be about when people die, about the differential presence of particular pathologies and about limitations placed on the life they lead while they are living it.

At the micro level, inequalities in health describe differences in the health state of the systems which are individual human beings but WHO turned us towards collectivities when it referred to 'peoples' rather than 'people'. As Carr-Hill and Chalmers-Dixon note:

> Whilst differences between individuals may well be interesting in themselves, they are only meaningful in terms of inequalities and inequities if these differences are linked to socio-economic status or some other dimension of differentiation. (2005: 156)

One obvious interpretation of the term 'peoples' is 'the populations of different nation states'.[21] So one definition of our population of collective cases is the set of nation states operationalised as those for which WHO has collected relevant data with health, operationalised through various aggregate measures, which in turn are derived from the aggregation of microdata describing the health states of individuals. In practice, we deal with other aggregates to examine inequalities within states.

The first two derive from the great biological and social divide among humans, gender. We can look at the health of men and women collectively, however defined, and typically health descriptors are organised by gender among all other aggregates for which we have measures. Another two, generally interrelated, principles of classification for the construction of aggregates are spatial – that is, descriptions of the health, however defined, of the populations of geographical areas at a variety of scales, and those based on some measure of social hierarchy. We often collect data organised by some description of 'ethnicity'. In some specific contexts we might regard religious adherence as a significant constitutor for health relevant aggregates. Geographical definitions are reasonably easy to construct. For the great majority of people who are not nomads they are based on 'home address', which can then be allocated to spatial units at varying scales. Measures of social hierarchy are much more varied and complex. In a wholly ascriptive society – for example, a pure caste society – one aspect of hierarchy is defined from birth. However, in most societies we want measures of social hierarchy which in some way address both of the dimensions which Max Weber described as 'class' and 'status' (1947). While Weber understood class in terms solely of command over market relations in terms of assets/income, other definitions include reference to position in a labour market, and in particular degree of authority and autonomy in work roles.[22] Status is a term used in relation to differences of social esteem, which are separate from monetary or monetisable resources. In principle, income and wealth are easily measurable. They are defined by money, which can be measured on a continuous scale, although in reality differences in monetary resources result in an ordinal hierarchy of kinds, albeit a decidedly fuzzy one. Status has been conventionally defined by occupation, or for non-workers by most recent occupation or occupation of a relative whose status is assumed to have a determinant power. Obviously, class definitions are related to traditional conceptions of capital, but we might think of status as related to elements of what is now generally referred to as 'social capital' – that is, personal attributes in terms of style, taste, education, networks of social connections and so on.

There are major questions as to how we operationalise class and status measures as attributes of individuals, which then become second-order issues as to how we organise those individuals into differentiated collectivities, but first let us consider the issue of time. Health is a product both of innate biological characteristics – the products of the complex interaction of individual genetic components – and of factors external to the individual but affecting that individual throughout their life course, including the prenatal element of that life course. However, most of our measures, both of health state and of the attributes we use to construct collectivities, are static. They are taken at a time point. We can, of course, attempt to reach back into the life course, so typically class differentiations in relation to length of life and cause of death are constructed by reaching back towards some sort of occupationally defined description of class based on most recent occupation (or occupation of relevant other) as stated on a death certificate. The health state of being dead is fine as a descriptor in terms of the dynamic trajectory of an individual system, but the class state is taken from a time point when that class state may have varied considerably throughout the life course of the individual, since occupations and relations change. A woman may have been the child of a female single-parent manual worker, become a clerical worker, first married another clerical worker, given up work, at some point returned to work, seen that marriage end, married a manager who through a management buyout became the owner of a large and successful enterprise, and then become an affluent widow after her second husband died. That is an account of the occupational and social role-defined class relations of a life course. We cannot adequately define it by a measurement at a single point in time, or rather cannot assess the causal power of class relations through a measurement taken at a single point in time. Equally, and again of significance in relation to the causes of health state, we move geographically in time, and actually places themselves change across time.[23] Any attribute of an individual may change, although gender and perhaps ethnicity are more stable than attributes defined by social hierarchies.

So far we have considered dynamism in terms of the potential for movement of individuals[24] across a life course around any classificatory system. However, we also have to consider potential changes in the nature of the classificatory systems themselves. In particular, we have to consider changes in the degree of differentiation of the elements of the classificatory system – that is, in the degree of inequality. Here we are dealing with changes of the kind measured for, say, incomes by a Gini coefficient.[25] Inequality is a variate attribute of whole social systems – not only of nation states but also of, for example, city regions – which has causal power in relation to the health states of individuals. Although usually examined by methods which relate continuous variates, it generally appears to have a threshold effect. So we have levels of inequality which are ranked classifications.

The issue of changes in classificatory systems themselves is general. Occupational rankings change through time. So, for example, in the contemporary UK the actual relative location of many public sector professional and semi-professional roles is being radically downgraded in the light of assaults on both remuneration (especially future pensions) and social status, which derive from government austerity measures. The social significance of level of education provides another example of the reality of changes in hierarchies. Although this may have an absolute effect across time – for example, in the relationship for women between completion of secondary education and numbers of pregnancies – more usually it changes in consequence of the upward movement of required level of education for occupational roles as the general level of education increases for successive age cohorts.[26]

The focus thus far has been on measuring health as an outcome for cases. Any discussion of health inequalities must also cover inequalities in the provision of health care, since this plainly has causal power in relation to inequalities in health outcomes, although that causal power always operates in complex interactions with other causal powers at all relevant levels. We cannot do this simply in terms of real expenditure on health care. This is poorly related to health outcomes because it is the organisation of health care systems as complex systems themselves in interaction with other complex systems at all levels (in particular, systems of housing provision and environmental protection) which has causal effects. A system that spends a great deal on end-of-life treatments for insured or otherwise affluent patients[27] may deliver poorly in terms of population health or even actually in terms of the health state across life of the patients who are the 'beneficiaries' of such expenditure. Just as social inequalities change over time, health service systems change over time and have effects through time.

The discussion of the relevance of degree of inequality across a social order in relation to health inequalities necessarily raises the issue of the causal powers of attributes of systems as a whole in relation to the microcomponents of the systems. Realist understanding acknowledges the causal powers of the whole over the part, and likewise recognises that subsets of parts have causal powers in relation to each other.

Inequality is described by comparisons across the microelements of a social system – for example, households described in terms of income. However, the causal power derives not from the attribute of those microelements but in the first instance from the relations among those elements and ultimately from the social mechanisms which generate those relations. So inequality in the contemporary UK is a product of the nature of post–industrial capitalism, which is in turn the product of specific human agency, including the agency of neoliberal ideological assertion within the academy. The system's character is made as it is by actors expressing their own material interests and those actors include the academic lackeys of the plutocracy, in particular those located in departments which peddle conventional (that is, not heterodox) economic theory.

Measuring in practice

The issues discussed thus far have been mostly to do with operationalisation (what are we measuring?) and casing (for what are we measuring it?), although we have also touched on issues of causality. We have discussed operationalisation and casing in relatively abstract terms, although in our view such an abstract discussion is an essential preliminary. Now we turn to the issue of how we measure in practical terms. What data and techniques can we deploy in order to assess health inequalities? To begin with the data, a range of sources have been used, and there is growing potential in the contemporary age of 'big data' to work in innovative ways which draw on the resources available in a world represented at all levels, including that of individuals, in electronic terms and also through time. The oldest data source is that vital (!) component of basic vital statistics, the death certificate. This has been used as the basis of measurement of health inequalities in the UK since the 1840s. Differential crude death rates actually drove service delivery, since a death rate above a threshold imposed a requirement to appoint a medical officer of health, which was a key factor in intervention. The death certificate remains a crucial data source, being used, for example, to construct occupationally related mortality tables. Obviously, death certificates deal in deaths – termination of human systems. Typically, they record age, address, cause of death and last occupation. In a prefiguring of the possibilities of big data it is possible to relate death certificates to information about individuals derived, for example, from censuses.

When we are dealing not with the termination of the system but with the actual health state of people who are still alive, then conventional data comes from two possible sources. One is any survey which includes questions asking respondents to describe their own health status. The other is the administrative records of elements of health provision systems at any level. Surveys typically ask people both to identify their current health state in broad descriptive terms and, for health-focused surveys, to provide information which enables categorisation of the degree of functionality of particular health subsystems – for example, assessing musculoskeletal health by asking respondents if they are capable of executing particular mobility-related tasks. This approach is particularly important for assessing differential mental health. Administrative records describe aspects of individual ill health including diagnoses, basic physiological measures, records of test results and records of treatments. It is these records in particular which are a key health source of 'big data'.

Big data is the most interesting potential source of information about health inequalities and factors relating to them. By the term 'big data' is meant the possible agglomeration of very large amounts of information about the attributes of individual people across time. We can explore big data because we have lots of information held in electronic form and we have data management tools which can put this data together across whole different domains. To say that there are issues of ethics and privacy in the construction and exploration of big datasets is to state the bleeding obvious. However, in principle,[28] the anonymisation of records can handle these issues. This would require an agreement that any records of a health system can be used for health-related research if they are anonymised. Rather than seeking individual consent, this could be established as a general principle. A clear difference should be established between the necessity for explicit informed consent to participation in research which involves active intervention on an individual and the use of anonymised records for epidemiological research.

Big data gives us very rich resources in terms of the information which could be useful for exploring health inequalities and, even more importantly, for hunting causal factors in the determination of those health inequalities. As with all uses of data we have to aggregate microdata for individuals in order to produce descriptions of health inequality. When we have limited information we can generally only do this for pre-established categories which are recorded on the data record. For example, when using UK death certificates we can only identify gender, location by postcode, and occupationally derived social class. However, the more information we have, the more subtly we can construct our classifications. With any reasonable survey we can construct categories using numerical typological procedures. We can classify according to any explicitly constructed principle, and even according to multiple principles, so we can explore the relationships among different systems of inequality. With big data collected over time we can in effect construct Poincaré sections which describe the position of our cases at discrete time points. We can map life trajectories. This enables us to do a lot more than construct health inequality tables. It has enormous importance for the exploration of the whole causal system in health, including the development of personalised treatment regimes, which assess interventions in relation not only to genome but also to life course (see Castellani and Castellani, 2003).

There is a degree of radical second-order empiricism involved in approaches of this kind. An extreme version would regard classifications as wholly emergent from the 'raw' big data, and there are data mining tools which can construct classifications without any input from pre-existing conceptions of what elements matter in relation to the construction of a classificatory system. However, when we choose what we classify by there is an input from pre-existing knowledge. A particularly fruitful approach is to classify entities on the basis of several different sets of classificatory principles and see how these relate to each other, but whenever we select variates as a basis for classification then we are deploying pre-existing knowledge, since we think that selection matters. It is particularly useful if we can classify across levels and especially when we can relate information about individuals to the character of the households of which they are members. This principle can be extended to any 'containing' level and particularly to geographical spaces – see Uprichard and Byrne (2007).

Conventional approaches to measuring health inequalities

As noted at the beginning of this chapter there is a substantial existing literature on measuring health inequalities. There is an excellent summary, which has not dated, to be found in Carr-Hill and Chalmers-Dixon's *Handbook of health inequalities measurement* (2005), prepared for the UK Public Health Observatories. This deals very well with conventional understandings of inequality and health and with the sources of data, although it does not deal with big data, understandably, since the development of a big data approach to health issues is very recent. A more recent summarising report is the EU's *Expert review and proposals for measuring health inequality* (Spinakis et al, 2011), which covers much the same ground. Characteristically for conventional discussions, considerable attention is devoted to the development of indices of health inequality. Indices in general are attempts to summarise multiple dimensions in a single continuous measure. The utility of this for comparison for administrative purposes is evident, but there is a serious question to be asked as to whether the construction of indices as scalars (continuous level of measurement) actually obscures important differences of kind, albeit of ordered kinds.[29]

A more extreme example of the issues that arise in developing measures of health inequality which purport to represent continuous differences is the development in the health economics literature of a series of attempts to import into the discussion the approaches developed by Atkinson (1970) for measurement of income inequalities. Erreygers (2013) adopts this approach. On the face of it, income inequality can properly be addressed by measurement at the continuous data level. After all, £50,000 is exactly one quarter of £200,000 and has one quarter of the purchasing power. However, if we think about the social implications of incomes of this level in the contemporary UK we can readily recognise that there is a qualitative difference, which is something different from the quantitative ratio between annual household incomes of £50,000 and £200,000. If we think of an annual household income of £100,000 then I think we will readily recognise that it gives access to many of the consumption/class behaviours characteristic of the household with an income of £200,000. For example, two children can be privately educated at both levels of income. If we consider a household with an annual income of £50,000 – that is, with the same ratio to the household with an annual income of £100,000 as that household has to the household with the income of £200,000 – then we can see that there are qualitative differences. Typical fees for private day schools in the UK are £9,000 per annum. That can be afforded for two children by the households with incomes of £100,000 and £200,000 but not by the household whose resources are solely represented by an annual income of £50,000. Those resources might stretch to one child in private education but two would be hard going. And households with annual incomes of £50,000 are well within the top quintile of UK household incomes, but are qualitatively different from those in the top half of the top decile. We have a difference of kind.

For all the reasons reviewed in the discussion of the nature of health understood as describing the state of individual human beings and thence of aggregates of human beings in terms of the state of complex systems, we cannot address health inequalities in continuous terms. Even if we think in terms of life expectancy, which on the face of it is a continuous variate, we should be able to see that is has different qualitative implications. For example, living to enjoy a well-funded retirement is qualitatively different from dying within a short period after retirement, an important mechanism by which male manual workers in particular fund the state pensions of higher social class non-manual workers. System states are categorical. We can certainly think of them in terms of ordered categories, but they are differences of kind, not of incremental degree. It is inequalities in system states which matter.

Probably the best and most appropriate conception of the health system state of an individual human being is to consider how we would operationalise the WHO definition in an age-appropriate fashion. Age appropriateness becomes very important when we have long lives, which take us into an inevitable state of differential functionality towards the end of them. We cannot do this simply in terms of calendar age. People of the same age, particularly in older life, have very different degrees of functionality. And what we think of as appropriate for an age changes over time. My partner and I, in our mid-sixties, were simultaneously amused and horrified when watching a 40-year-old episode of *The Likely Lads* to find people of our age now presented as really old, but when we were in our twenties most working class people of that age *were* old in terms of physical and social functionality. While 60 may be the new 40, 80 is probably old and 90 definitely is still old.

For aggregates what matters is the degree of inequality among the aggregates, and it is necessary to reiterate that this must be understood in terms of threshold effects. This is a matter of causality. The relationship between inequalities among aggregates in terms of complexes causal to health state is not linear. The health consequences become much more severe for inequality at thresholds. However, whereas the health states of individuals are categories, and therefore differences among individuals are categorical differences, when we deal with aggregates these categorical differences become smoothed out so we cannot see them in the same way. This is why conventional measures of health inequalities among social categories rely on simple indices in the form of percentage of the category dying prematurely or being incapacitated in some aspect of health state. These are useful, but they conceal differences within categories and offer us less of a clue to actual causal processes. There are differences within social categories as well as among social categories, and big data offers us the possibility of identifying these differences and using them to develop causal models which do not assign all the causal power simply to the category itself.

We can categorise extensively using big data and then explore the relationships of categories with health outcomes, taking account of significant social categories themselves. The most powerful and historically significant social category has always been social class because it is precisely founded, however measured, in some conception of hierarchically ordered social inequalities. Gender plainly has a substantial biological component but its social expression also reflects structural inequality between men and women. Ethnicity is the most plastic category, but in societies where ethnic identity and classification have been part of structures of inequality themselves, then of course it can and does have causal powers, however complex these are in expression. It is tempting, and in important ways it is not wrong, to assign causal powers simply to these very powerful social categories precisely because they are, to use Byrne's (2002) description, powerful traces of the unequal structuring of the social systems as a whole. As gross descriptors they matter because the presentation of inequalities in terms of them has political power.

If we simply 'classify' rather than establish our categories on the basis of some understanding of the determinant processes in relation to structures of inequality – class for capitalism, gender for patriarchy, ethnicity for racism/colonialism – then our accounts can be accused of being of the form that C. Wright Mills derided as 'abstracted empiricism' (Mills, 1962). However, classification has value for descriptive exploration and can reveal the ways in which the great differentiating principles of class, gender and ethnicity actually interact in determining social outcomes and, in particular, health outcomes. Here, it is important to emphasise that the word 'determine' is being used in the sense suggested by Williams (1980). That is to say it sets limits to a range of possibilities rather than specifying particular and exact outcomes which always occur. Even if we construct complex categories that correspond to the locations of cases within the possibility state which includes all possible causal factors as specifying dimensions, then we will find not exact points indicating outcomes but rather clouds of cases within an attractor set (see Byrne and Callaghan, 2013). Nonetheless, these categories will be sufficiently distinctive to be useful both for description and as a starting point in relation to the development of transformative interventions. Dyer's work (2006) on the trajectories of cases passing through a forensic psychiatric custody diversion service demonstrates how this can be done using individual level data.

To conclude this discussion, let us consider the most common traditional level of focus of public health interventions, at the level of some spatial unit – usually either an administrative/political locality or in relation to internal spatial differentiation within such a locality.

All the remarks about the use of big data apply to these levels as well, although of course the 'big' here refers to numbers of measurements of traces of these systems rather than to the number of individual cases in the datasets. Moreover, through the use of administrative records and standard sources of secondary data – in particular, censuses – we can achieve a great deal in terms of description as a basis for classifying. Blackman et al (2011b) used this kind of approach to considerable effect in developing an exploratory causal account of different trajectories in closing health inequalities across Spearhead local health areas in England.

Conclusion

Measurement matters in order to describe, but it also matters, using the title of Cartwright's (2007b) book, for *Hunting causes and using them*. It is plainly evident that the great structural forces of inequality – a capitalist social order, patriarchy, racism and post-colonialism – are causal, and that policies directed at them matter a great deal. Equalities legislation and practices can address patriarchy and racism/post-colonialism as well as any other identity-constituted inequalities. Class is a harder matter, since addressing inequalities predicated on it always constitutes a challenge to the social structures which emerge from capitalism. However, even within a capitalist order, taking account of Westergaard's very clearly specified 'limits to reform' (1978), changes are possible. General promotion of equality through the use of benefits and taxation and, above all, the empowerment of trade unions matters. Specific policies matter. The massive reduction in the social salience of TB in the UK owed more to the programme of council house building than any other intervention, including the development and refinement of curative programmes. The big things matter.

But so do the details – the kind of complex associations which can be established through careful measurement and review of data. The identification of asbestos as a major source of morbidity stands as an excellent example of the establishment of a simple and sufficient cause.[30] Lots of causes are complex, and while necessary are not sufficient. Understanding health inequalities and the determinants of health inequalities in terms of intersected complex systems at a variety of levels can help us delve into these and can help to identify ways in which interventions might make a difference. As always, this will only happen if the major structural determinants and, in particular, inequalities of power are always in our sights for action.

Part Two
Health inequalities in England

FIVE

A history of health inequalities in England

Introduction

Part Two of this book provides a fuller account of the nature and extent of health inequalities in England. It also reviews the policies that have been developed to address such inequalities and their impact in recent years, to the extent that it is possible to attribute causal relationships in a field as complex as that being considered here. Our interest in policy is twofold: it includes both the design of interventions to combat inequalities and the governance arrangements designed to implement them. In this chapter we concentrate on providing a historical overview of policy and implementation in the period from the first statutory intervention in health in 1848 to the introduction of a universal health service in 1948 and the more recent initiatives to address health inequalities under the Labour government of 1997 to 2010. The chapter reviews the evidence for the nature and extent of health inequalities today and analyses the policies of the current Coalition government towards health inequalities and the governance of public health more generally.

The early public health movement

Two of the most important events in the history of health and health services for the population of the UK are separated by exactly 100 years. While 1848 marked the passage of the first Public Health Act, 1948 was the year in which the National Health Service (NHS) first opened its doors. From July that year, access to health services was no longer to be determined by inequalities of income and wealth, albeit leavened by charity or means tests: instead, it was intended that comprehensive services should be available to all, free at the point of use. The early development of public policy on health inequalities was not, however, initially understood in terms of promoting universal access to health care; nor, indeed, was it contemplated that the state should have any kind of role in extending access to services providing treatment and care. Rather, when the responsibility of government for the health of the population first came to be recognised, it was conceived in terms of initiatives and interventions to improve public health but not to provide personal medical services. In addition, while the modern history of health inequalities tends to be associated with the Black Report of 1980, public health policy and its response to variations in health outcomes have a much longer history. Indeed, public health policy long pre-dated the NHS; it began when high rates of death and disease seemed part of the natural order and the notion that the state should take action on behalf of its citizens to reduce premature or avoidable deaths would have been unthinkable if not incomprehensible. Hamlin and Sheard (1998) note that by the early nineteenth century the state in Britain and other parts of Europe did respond to threats to population health at times of 'unusual disease' (epidemics, especially of cholera and typhoid), only to fall back into inaction once the danger had passed. By contrast, 'normal disease – infant mortality of more than 50% in inner-city wards, annual mortality of over 30/1000 in some towns – prompted no such reactions'. This lack of consistency in state responses to health and disease started to change during the 1840s, and the acceptance began to develop that the state should be the proactive and statutory 'guarantor of standards of health and environmental quality and (provide) means for local units of government to make the structural changes to meet those standards' (Hamlin and Sheard, 1998: 587). Thus, the development of the public health function, rather than the provision of publicly funded health services, was the first area of substantial intervention by the state. Indeed, as we have already indicated, the first Public Health Act of 1848 preceded the establishment of the NHS by a full century.

Two aspects of the 1848 Act should be highlighted here. First, it originated in the well-known and determined efforts of Edwin Chadwick to establish and conduct an inquiry into 'the sanitary conditions of the labouring population' (Chadwick, 1842). What may be less well remembered is that Chadwick's interest in this issue arose from his responsibilities for implementing the Poor Law Amendment Act 1834, of which he was himself the principal author and which aimed to deter applications for poor relief. His concern to reduce costs wherever possible led him to be wary of approaches which dealt predominantly with the symptoms of poverty. Instead, he recognised that efficiency and what we would now call better value or cost–effectiveness necessitated a focus on identifying and addressing the causes of poverty. At this point in his investigations, he pinpointed the death of male breadwinners from infectious diseases as a principal driver of family poverty.

His solution was to stress the importance of supplying constant clean water supplies and the efficient removal of sewage. This approach was well founded as far as it went, but in reality it neglected the claims of poor law officers and other medical officers that poverty and the harsh enforcement of the Poor Law were themselves what we would now describe as 'causes of the causes' of disease and premature deaths. However, as Hamlin and Sheard point out, Chadwick suppressed 'the other half of the vicious circle – that deprivation might itself cause the disease that left so many dependent ...' (1998: 588). As we will show below, this was not to be the only occasion when politically inconvenient evidence about the relationship between poverty and ill health was to be discarded or ignored.

A second feature of the 1848 Act and early debates about public health, which also continues to be of relevance today, relates to issues of governance and the balance between individual and collective responsibilities. On the one hand, questions were raised about the balance between the rights of individual property owners and the powers of a potentially dictatorial state and its inflexible bureaucracy to insist upon and manage sanitary reform. On the other hand, the respective roles of central government and local units of government were also a matter of debate and controversy. Ultimately, the 1848 Act settled these disputes in favour of voluntarism and localism: groups of local ratepayers (at least 10% of the total) could request the establishment of an elected local board of health to improve water supplies and sanitation. Similarly, local boards could appoint 'medical officers of health', but this was not compulsory. However, in areas with high death rates (23 per 1000 population and above), a local board could be imposed from the centre by a newly established General Board of Health. The overall tenor of the Act was, in Hamlin and Sheard's (1998) terms, one of 'facilitating' rather than 'forcing', in a context where public health legislation became 'an instrument for local democracy', albeit that of upper-middle-class men in the towns.

Chadwick had had to campaign hard for the legislation, and both he and the General Board of Health, of which he became the commissioner, were to remain unpopular with those opposed to what they saw as the unjustified infringement of private interests by an overbearing state. Ultimately he was forced from office, and progress in individual areas depended on local motivation and leadership. Nonetheless, local boards and their officers, surveyors from the outset and medical officers of health where local people wished, began to promote a range of sanitary, environmental and (later) housing improvements which came to be recognised, together with improved living standards, as key contributors to reductions in mortality.

Under the Sanitary Acts of 1866–70, local authorities became responsible for the provision of sewers, water and street cleaning and had to appoint sanitary inspectors. Subsequent developments were accelerated and extended by the work of a Royal Sanitary Commission (1869–1871), which led to the establishment of the Local Government Board in 1871, together with the Public Health Acts of 1872 and 1875. The latter consolidated previous acts into a single set of powers and duties, while the former legislated for the creation of a local governance system for improving the health of the public through the establishment of sanitary committees and the (now compulsory) appointment of a local medical officer of health. Such officers had already played a leading role in pioneering towns and cities in environmental improvements to combat infectious disease conditions. They were to become key local actors in championing better health, while the local sanitary committees evolved into a broader system of local government. Indeed, the post-1848 local boards of health proved to be fundamental building blocks in the development of the modern system of multi-purpose democratically elected local authorities. In short, the 1848 Act was a starting point for a national structure of local government as much as for a comprehensive national health service.

These two development paths were brought together when a Royal Commission sat from 1905 to 1909 to review the future of the Poor Law. A 'minority report' from the Commission advocated a unified medical service within local government. Although this recommendation was not adopted, local authorities did take over responsibility for poor law infirmaries (and workhouses) in 1929, and a number of city councils began a substantial programme of developing municipal hospitals. Although they had been given this power under the Public Health Act 1875, only three such hospitals had been built before 1930. By 1938, however, local authorities provided 75,000 general acute beds and the London County Council was arguably the biggest hospital authority in the world, with as many beds as the national network of voluntary hospitals (Timmins, 1995: 106). With the advent of the NHS, all these different categories of hospital were nationalised and local government responsibilities reverted to public health and the development of services in the community, though general practitioners (GPs) remained a separate branch of the service as independent contractors.

A health service for everyone

The establishment of a national health service a century after the first Public Health Act is, rightly, seen as the culmination of a campaign during the first half of the twentieth century to secure universal access to a comprehensive set of health services of uniformly high quality across the whole country. Comprehensive in terms of geography, provision and population coverage, it also aimed to remove financial barriers to access by being funded overwhelmingly from general taxation and free at the point of access. Framed in these terms, it is little surprise that the NHS became, and remains, one of the most popular and trusted institutions in the country, widely perceived to be the principal guarantor of individual health and increasing life expectancy among the population as a whole. Yet, as we show elsewhere in this book, it has failed to eradicate inequalities in health outcomes. Life expectancy at birth varies by as much as seven years between different local authority areas. Similar inequalities are also evident in the experience of healthy life expectancy, with a difference of 17.5 years for men and 15.5 years for women between the highest and lowest local authority areas (ONS, 2014a). The social gradient in health applies, therefore, to the extent to which life is added to years as well as years to life.

These are major shortcomings in a supposedly universal service based on need rather than geography or economic status. This apparent contradiction between universal access to health services and persistent inequalities in health outcomes is a concern of this book. How is it that substantial, and growing, inequalities in health outcomes can exist more than six decades after financial barriers to access were abolished and comprehensive health services were introduced for the whole population? We can explain this apparent contradiction at two levels. First, not all local health systems are the same: variations exist in the availability of services of a similar range and quality. Even more significantly, 'poorer areas tend to have worse health services' (Baggott, 2004: 65). Patterns of access contain many complexities, including variations by geography and presentation for treatment. However, Tudor Hart's (1971) 'inverse care law', which suggests that the availability of good medical care varies inversely with the need for it, remains relevant as an explanation for socioeconomic differences in access to the NHS.

The second level of explanation for the existence of health inequalities within a universal and longstanding NHS is more fundamental still, with its roots in the logic model which dominated its initial design and continuing operation since 1948. Over time, it has become a commonplace to suggest that the NHS is a misnomer for what should more accurately be labelled a national illness service (NIS) or national sickness service (NSS). Ministerial responsibilities under the NHS Act 1946 included the prevention of disease and promotion of health, but these duties have, in practice, remained secondary to those involved in promoting and securing the delivery of a comprehensive health service. In the first decade of this century only around 4% of the NHS budget was spent on preventing illness and promoting health (NAO, 2013) The dominant model shaping the allocation of resources in the NHS and underpinning its operating logic was and remains one which responds to problems presented by patients in their individual consultations with medical practitioners. It is for this reason that we prefer the terminology of 'universal personal medical services' to describe the principal offer the NHS was designed to make. If only implicitly, the role of the state came to be defined in terms of funding 'health for all' through a diagnosis, treatment and recovery service for those experiencing illness and disability. Thus, the campaigns for comprehensive and universal health care were understood more in terms of securing 'equal' access to a comprehensive range of personal medical services, free at the point of delivery, rather than of enabling the population to enjoy similar periods of healthy life expectancy, irrespective of income, place of residence or other socioeconomic factors.

The failure to end health inequalities by removing financial barriers to personal medical services should not, however, diminish the critical importance of this feature of the NHS to those otherwise unable to meet the costs of care. Nor should it diminish the contribution of services free at the point of delivery to the removal of the catastrophic impact of major illness on personal finances, quality of life or life expectancy. We should also recall that a comprehensive health service 'without a charge on treatment at any point' (Beveridge, 1942: 14) was one of the 'three assumptions' on which Beveridge based his plan for social security and the attack on 'Want' (the two other assumptions being universal family allowances and full employment). Thus, 'free health care' was itself seen as necessary to prevent poverty and sustain economic activity through a healthy workforce. A failure to value and sustain such features of the NHS into the future will leave us poorer as a society as well as individuals. Even so, we should be cautious of equating the necessary removal of up-front financial barriers to diagnosis and treatment with an operating model which is sufficient to reduce inequalities in healthy life expectancy. To develop the latter we would need to understand and target the underlying causes of variations in life expectancy. Investing resources in immediate and universal access to medical services, the principal operating model for the NHS, can still be seen as a diversion from health for all as opposed to health (medical) care for all. To that extent, the NHS is a category error of the highest order: it can be seen as a diversion from identifying not only 'the causes of the causes' of disease and disability but also the socially and economically structured patterns of such determinants of health and wellbeing. It is as though the public health revolution of the second half of the nineteenth and the early twentieth century was deemed to have completed its course, and all that remained was to patch up those on whom the chance and arbitrary forces of nature had visited poor health and disability.

To some extent, the limitations of such a logic model are demonstrated by the flawed expectations of NHS founders and the subsequent history of the NHS. Aneurin Bevan himself envisaged that once the backlog of untreated conditions had been cleared, following the introduction of 'free' services, both demand and costs would fall (Timmins, 1995: 132). While it might take time to ensure that the necessary staffing and financial resources were equally available throughout the country, these were essentially technical issues of allocative efficiency, which could be addressed by developing services to meet observed demand. By removing the financial barriers to treatment, free personal health services would promote early access to treatment, and investment in the NHS would bring its own return as it succeeded in improving the nation's health. This belief was not challenged effectively until the 1956 Guillebaud Report, which, in arguing for increased investment in the service, dryly commented that 'it is still sometimes assumed that the health service can and should be self-limiting, in the sense that its own contribution to the national health will limit the demands upon it to a volume that can be fully met. This, at least for the present, is an illusion' (cited in Timmins, 1995: 207). The reasons this belief has remained an illusion are many but include developments in medicine and associated technologies that were unforeseen in 1948 and make so many more tests and treatments possible. In addition, the pattern of disease has changed with the substantial growth in long-term conditions and multi-morbidity characteristic of ageing populations and greater economic affluence. Managing the resulting disabilities, restricting their deterioration and providing continuing support are more characteristic of the NHS today than the classic pattern of episodic illness and self-limiting medical interventions which formed the paradigm for its operation in 1948.

Summary discussion

During the Victorian heyday of public health, sanitary reform and concerns about the 'health of towns' framed understandings of health and of the necessary objects of public investment. The Public Health Act of 1848 was significant in a number of ways. First, it sought to address the most substantial threats to health – infectious diseases like cholera and typhoid. Second, it proposed interventions based on evidence its advocates had collected about the causes of those diseases, namely clean and continuous water supplies and separate sanitation systems. Third, it led to the beginnings of a rudimentary organisational infrastructure for a system of shared central and local responsibilities. Over the century between the first Public Health Act and the beginning of the NHS, however, this 'public health paradigm' was superseded by one organised around the centrality of personal medical services. The contribution of the latter grew with the recognition and regulation of medical practitioners under the General Medical Act 1858, together with the development of poor law infirmaries and voluntary hospitals funded as charitable foundations. During the first half of the twentieth century, it came to dominate understanding and expectations of what a publicly funded service would look like and 'do'. As a result, it provided the principal operating model for the NHS and has dominated its development over more than six decades. From the early 1960s onwards, it was built around the development, for every part of the country, of a district general hospital (which absorbed the bulk of public investment), to which GP and community health services principally played second fiddle.

An implicit underlying assumption of the NHS was that removing financial barriers to accessing comprehensive personal medical services would enable the levelling up of health outcomes. The improved availability of such services for the population as a whole would lead to better outcomes for all. In practice, as we have seen, improvements in health and life expectancy have not been universally enjoyed: there is a marked and currently growing social gradient in healthy life expectancy. We have suggested that, while variations in access to universally high-quality services may help to explain the persistence of unequal outcomes, a more fundamental problem lies in a medical model which, by definition, focuses on identifying and responding to symptoms more than causes. Since the latter are primarily rooted in social and economic factors whose distribution and influence tend to be concentrated on the more disadvantaged people and places in our society, personal medicine can never make more than a partial contribution to the levelling up of rates of healthy life expectancy. As a result, the universalisation of health services has proved to be only a partial response to the structural causes of health inequalities. In terms of the theoretical framework introduced in Chapter Two, personal medicine should be seen as a linear operating model incapable of dealing with all the socioeconomic factors which cause and sustain inequalities in health and life expectancy. In effect, it is a tame solution to a wicked problem. To the extent that public policy and spending priorities are dominated by this model, their ability to reduce health inequalities will remain seriously compromised. We return to this issue in the final chapter.

Emerging challenges to the personal medicine paradigm

The 1970s marked the beginning of a series of challenges to the personal medicine paradigm, which continue today. These challenges were of two different kinds: first, a challenge to the perception that personal medicine was actually responsible for increasing life expectancy to the extent that public opinion and professional interests generally recognised; and second, a challenge to the effectiveness of personal medicine on its own terms. The initial challenge was posed in Thomas McKeown's 1976 Rock Carling Fellowship monograph on the role of medicine. By reviewing historical trends in mortality rates, he demonstrated that the greatest reductions in mortality came before the introduction of new drugs and surgical procedures underlying personal medicine. As a result, he concluded that:

> medical science and services are misdirected, and society's investment in health is not well used, because they rest on an erroneous assumption about the basis of human health. It is assumed that the body can be regarded as a machine whose protection from disease and its effects depends primarily on internal intervention. The approach has led to indifference to the external influences and personal behaviour which are the predominant determinants of health. (McKeown, 1976: xiv)

Baggott (2004) identifies a number of subsequent challenges to McKeown's thesis, which suggest that he did not give sufficient weight to the contribution of modern medicine in terms of saving lives and improving quality of life. Nevertheless, the Royal Commission on the NHS of 1979 supported McKeown's approach, noting that historically the biggest advances in health status were the result of clean water and better housing. Accordingly, it concluded that 'on the basis of past experience, a substantial improvement in national and community health is more likely to be achieved by preventive measures' (Parliament, 1979: para 5.3). Klein highlights the public expenditure implications of this conclusion, noting the Royal Commission's finding that 'international comparisons do not suggest that greater expenditure automatically leads to better health ... and it is at least arguable that the improvement in the health of the nation would be greater if extra resources were, for example, devoted to better housing' (1995: 120–1). Thus, as the 1970s drew to a close, the personal medicine paradigm was being subjected to a form of scrutiny which represented a new departure in the history of the NHS, as authoritative voices questioned what had become the conventional wisdom that investments in the NHS necessarily provided the only or most cost-effective route to better health outcomes.

The role of medicine came under scrutiny from other directions, especially of how effective it was in its own terms. Part of McKeown's critique was that medicine had been allowed to be judged on 'its own valuation' of its worth and contribution to health and society. Cochrane (1972) asserted that the evidence base for much medical practice was underdeveloped, which led to most treatment-related decisions not being based on a systematic review of clinical evidence. He advocated the development of evidence-based practice, based on systematic reviews and the adoption of randomised control trials (RCTs) to provide rigorous assessments of the efficiency and effectiveness of specific interventions. He also argued that the hospital was not necessarily the optimal setting for treatment and care, pointing out that primary and home care settings might be as or more effective and efficient. His work was important in demonstrating that a universal service did not necessarily guarantee universal standards of clinical outcome or resource utilisation. The goal of reducing unjustified and unjustifiable variations in individual clinical practice or service organisation remains a high priority, reflected in, for example, current priorities to improve patient safety, reduce 'unnecessary' admissions/ lengths of stay and develop – through the National Institute for Health and Care Excellence (NICE) – guidelines for clinical practice and prescribing.

Cochrane led a technical challenge to medicine, arguing that it should embrace the scientific method more systematically and adopt evidence-based practice. His legacy is reflected in the widespread view that RCTs represent the 'gold standard' for evaluation (though we drew attention to their limitations in Chapter Two) and in the development of the Cochrane Collaboration to promote international collaborations to conduct systematic reviews of clinical trials by specialty. A more sociological and fundamental challenge to medicine came from Ivan Illich (1975; 1976) in his books *Limits to medicine* and *Medical nemesis*. He not only shared a similar view to McKeown's that the role of medicine had been overvalued in explanations of improvements in life expectancy and the quality of life but also claimed that it could be positively harmful. He introduced the term 'iatrogenesis' (literally 'doctor-generated') to describe illness produced by medical activity. This phenomenon was identified as having three dimensions:

- clinical iatrogenesis, referring to errors, accidents, malpractice and side effects of diagnostic and treatment procedures;
- social iatrogenesis, resulting from the medicalisation of more aspects of life experiences, including the focus by professionals on disease rather than health which we have already identified; and
- cultural iatrogenesis, according to which medicine offers a technical solution to man-made pain, reinforcing dependency on medicine and diverting attention from social and political causes of ill health.

We can see elements of all three of these dimensions in contemporary debates about the NHS, including concerns about patient safety as exemplified by the Mid Staffordshire enquiry; arguments about how extensively statins should be prescribed compared with encouraging lifestyle change; unease about the management of death and dying, ranging from the 'artificial' prolongation of life – as seen to be illustrated by debates about assisted suicide and the 'right to die' – to the inappropriate utilisation of end-of-life protocols such as the Liverpool Care Pathway; and the extent to which public policy should switch resources to prevention and from health services to social care or to moderating the impact of the social and economic determinants of health. From the perspective of the historical overview around which this chapter is organised, however, the wider point we wish to emphasise is that, from the 1970s onwards, the personal medicine paradigm has been subjected to a series of critiques from the different standpoints of history, scientific method, economics and sociology.

These challenges have exposed more clearly the conceptual foundations and operating model on which the NHS was largely based. In the process, its limitations have become clearer and its presumed benefits less taken for granted. It remains the dominant influence on understandings of the purpose and form of interventions to improve health, but it is more vulnerable to scrutiny than previously. Recent revelations about patient safety and poor care have contributed to a climate of disquiet about a service whose role in saving lives has hitherto placed it almost beyond criticism in some quarters. There are risks of an overcorrection taking place in policy makers' perceptions of the NHS or of the medical model's limitations being too readily interpreted as limitations of universal, state-funded services. However, it may also be that greater space is opening up for a more open public debate about the extent to which a different balance between personal medicine and public health is appropriate. This debate has been made both more necessary, and more possible, by the accumulation of evidence that health inequalities have been intensifying rather than diminishing, notwithstanding the provision of universal health services free at the point of delivery. This is not to argue that the medical model has no role but to contend that we need to understand its limitations, especially in solving largely social problems such as health inequalities.

The origins of contemporary health inequalities policy: the Black and Acheson Reports

A renewed focus on health inequalities began to emerge during the 1970s, the same decade in which the challenges to personal medicine also began to emerge and gain ground. The modern concerns about the socioeconomic determinants of health and their unequal impact on health and life expectancy are generally traced back to the Black Report (1980). This document was one of two reports on health inequalities – the second being the Acheson Report (Acheson, 1998) – whose publication effectively marked the defeat of the Callaghan Labour government in 1979 and the election of Tony Blair's New Labour government in 1997. In between, the Conservative governments of Margaret Thatcher and John Major first sought to 'bury' the whole concept of inequalities in health and only later accepted the legitimacy of exploring the significance of what were officially termed 'variations' in health.

The 1974–9 government had expressed a commitment to developing a greater emphasis on the prevention of disease and promotion of health. In 1976, it published a consultation document on priorities for health and social services, the first ever comprehensive statement of priorities and plans for allocating resources between and within the NHS and personal social services. From our perspective, the document was significant in endorsing the challenge to medical practice which had been posed by Cochrane; it particularly focused on identifying opportunities to improve cost–effectiveness by reducing variations in clinical practice and shifting the balance between hospital and community care. This approach was one of the first to seek to bring individual clinical practice within a resource-management framework and, as such, to challenge medical practitioners' traditional claim to clinical autonomy, the freedom to base individual practice on the exercise of independent professional judgement. The document was accompanied by another Green Paper, which also reflected the influence of the challenges to the personal medicine paradigm outlined above. This document – *Prevention and health: Everybody's business* (DHSS, 1976) was the first such NHS policy review covering prevention and marked the beginning of a re-emphasis on the importance of factors other than medicine in improving health. Thus, it endorsed the view that in the past improvements in health and life expectancy owed more to public health than personal medicine. For the future, it emphasised that continuing improvements would depend on encouraging people to take responsibility for their own health and change behaviours associated with ill health and premature death. Changes to diet, smoking cessation, more exercise, reducing alcohol and drug abuse were among areas identified as health-promoting behaviours. The following year saw the publication of the White Paper *Prevention and Health* (DHSS, 1977), but its tangible initiatives were largely focused on funding the expansion of health education. Baggot provides a useful perspective on its approach: 'interventionist measures were avoided, for fear of upsetting commercial interests and the public, whom the politicians believed would resent attempts to regulate lifestyles. Aside from an increase in health education spending, Government was reluctant to provide extra resources to encourage prevention and divert resources from high technology medicine' (2004: 334). This more limited focus on education and behavioural change was to be a characteristic of policy and politics under successive governments, and the more radical elements of the challenge to personal medicine were not followed up in practice.

The Black Report, 1980

A different route to improving health and life expectancy was presented, but immediately sidelined, through the Black Report on inequalities in health. Both its commissioning and publication are themselves important elements in the rebirth of public health. Its origins lay in an open letter from a Master's student of community medicine at Nottingham University in 1976 to David Ennals, the Secretary of State for Health. The student, Richard Wilkinson (who was to become an important contributor to more recent policy analysis on the impact of inequalities on health status), argued that – notwithstanding the introduction of the NHS – the gap in health status between upper and lower classes appeared to be two or three times higher in the 1970s than in the 1930s and 1940s. He also suggested that this trend was one that Ennals would want not only to halt but also to reverse (Wilkinson, 1976). This appears to have prompted Ennals to set up an inquiry chaired by Sir Douglas Black, Chief Scientist at the Department of Health (DH), with the following broad objectives:

- to assemble available information about the differences in health status among the social classes and about factors which might contribute to these, including relevant data from other industrial countries;
- to analyse this material in order to identify possible causal relationships, to examine the hypotheses that have been formulated and the testing of them, and to assess the implications for policy; and
- to suggest what further research should be initiated (Black, 1980: Introduction).

The Report was completed following a change of government, and was received less than enthusiastically by the new Conservative administration led by Margaret Thatcher. Indeed, it is remembered almost as much for its reception as for its detailed content. The document was released over the 1980 August bank holiday weekend, with little publicity and in a cyclostyle[31] edition of 260 copies, rather than as a printed government report published by HMSO. It was accompanied by a brief letter from the Secretary of State, Patrick Jenkins, which stated:

> I must make it clear that additional expenditure on the scale which could result from the report's recommendations – the amount involved could be upward of £2 billion a year – is quite unrealistic in present or any foreseeable economic circumstances, quite apart from any judgements that may be formed of the effectiveness of such expenditure in dealing with the problems identified. I cannot, therefore, endorse the Group's recommendations. (cited in Townsend et al, 1992: 16–17) The Black Report found that, despite improvements in overall health, inequalities had grown in

the 20-year period up to the early 1970s covered by its analysis. In particular, it identified that:

- mortality rates for men and women in social classes I and II had declined substantially but those for social classes IV and V had deteriorated in relation to the top two social classes;mortality rates for class V were twice those for class I;
- gender, as well as class inequalities were evident: men had higher death rates than women across all social classes (Black, 1980).

The Report recognised that explaining the persistence and growth of such inequalities was not a straightforward matter. In fact, it identified four potential explanations for the relationship between health and inequality: the social selection explanation, the artefact explanation, cultural and behavioural explanations and structural and material explanations. Black's account of them has been usefully summarised elsewhere in the following terms.

- The social selection explanation. In this view illness is not the result of low income and poverty, but the cause of them. Healthy people are more likely to be upwardly mobile, while those who are ill become downwardly mobile.
- The artefact explanation. This view states that statistical comparisons between social classes tend to exaggerate the extent of inequality because the working class (the poor health class) is shrinking while the middle class (the good health class) is expanding.
- Cultural and behavioural explanations. Unequal health stems from differences in the behaviour of people from different classes: working class people have worse health because they are more likely to engage in health-damaging behaviour, such as smoking, drinking alcohol, etc.
- Structural and material explanations. These see social inequality and material conditions as the cause of health inequalities. These include poverty and material deprivation stemming from unemployment, low income, bad housing conditions, polluted environments, and unhealthy or dangerous working conditions. Low

> social position is associated with a lack of control over one's life and with higher levels of stress and thus poor health. (http://socialscience.stow.ac.uk/rab/hnc_health/modelsofhealth.htm accessed on 23rd July 2013)

The Black Report itself concluded that the most relevant evidence came from the 'materialist' or 'structuralist' explanation. Indeed, the artefact and social selection explanations were barely mentioned in the subsequent Acheson Report or Marmot Review as, by this stage, the research that had been undertaken on health inequalities meant that these explanations were largely no longer considered realistic (Bambra et al, 2011). The Black Report further concluded that:

> some of the evidence on class inequalities in health is adequately understood in terms of specific features of the socioeconomic environment: features (such as accidents at work, overcrowding, smoking) which are strongly class-related in Britain and also have clear aetiological significance ... [however] there is undoubtedly much which cannot be understood in terms of the impact of so specific factors. Much, we feel, can only be understood in terms of the more diffuse consequences of the class structure: poverty, work conditions (and what we termed the social division of labour), and deprivation in its various forms. (Black, 1980: 6.93)

As Blane (1991: 126) highlights, the Black Report concluded that class differences in mortality were primarily due to the combined effect of class differences in exposure to a wide range of factors which promoted health or caused disease. However, the report emphasised that the health service itself played only a marginal role in causing inequalities in health (Oliver, 2008). If we revert to the lens provided by complexity theory, we can see that the Black Report stated that the causes of health inequalities were to be understood within a whole system perspective, in which individual elements were interdependent, dynamic and non-linear:

> It is this acknowledgement of the complex nature of the explanation of health inequalities – involving access to and use of the health services; specific issues in other areas of social policy; and more general features of class, material

inequality, and deprivation – which informs and structures the recommendations we make. (Black, 1980: 6.94)

The report included 37 recommendations to reduce health inequalities, which focused particularly on action to mitigate the structural and material causes it had identified. These included increases in child benefits, more comprehensive services for children under five, improvements to housing, free school meals, shifting resources to health and social care services in the community and improving prevention measures such as programmes to reduce smoking and increase physical activity. It also argued that 'greater co-ordination between Government Departments in the administration of health related policies is required ... Local counterparts of national coordinating bodies also need to be established' (Black, 1980).

As we have seen, central government did not respond positively to any of these recommendations. Nathanson reminds us that 'The Lancet described the government's reaction as "frosty" in its total rejection of the report's recommendations to reallocate and increase financial resources directed towards – among other goals – abolishing child poverty. Clearly, the Conservative Government of the day had no wish to own – i.e., acknowledge responsibility for solving – health inequalities' (2010: 275). Illsley notes that 'Black's recommendations would have presented problems for any government as it contained a 130-page "wish list" and was therefore, given the UK's economic difficulties at the time, "a report waiting to be rejected"' (cited in Bambra et al, 2011: 4). As a result, the impact on policy was minimal and, as Timmins highlights, it 'launched the start of a decade of uncomfortable and ultimately unsustainable denials by government that health had anything to do with socio-economic conditions' (1995: 380). However, Oliver (2008) contends that the Black Report was significant in other respects, and especially in terms of stimulating research among those in opposition to the Thatcher government's perspective on health inequalities.

By 1987, however, the government's views had shifted at least to the extent of taking greater interest in the potential of prevention through the publication of the White Paper *Promoting better health* (DHSS, 1987). Indeed, Klein argues that this document showed that 'the Thatcher administration had become converted, with some enthusiasm, to the cause of health prevention ... [and] to promote health and prevent illness' (1995: 167–8). The Conservative election manifesto for that year's general election had contained six guiding policies on health, one of which was 'the prevention of avoidable illness and the promotion of good health'. Klein (1995: 168) points out that this newfound enthusiasm for health promotion was at first puzzling, as prevention had tended to be an interest of the left. Indeed, health promotion tended to be associated in the minds of many Conservatives with the nanny state interfering with the way in which people run their lives – for example taking more exercise or giving up smoking. The government's conversion appears to have had two drivers: AIDS and money. The absence of a known cure for the former inevitably placed a higher priority on prevention. Within the Department of Health and Social Security (DHSS), the AIDS epidemic created a new constituency of support for preventive strategies and strengthened the influence of Donald Acheson, the Chief Medical Officer. The only policy instruments that appeared to be available were traditional public health tools, and the government committed itself to a major campaign of public health education covering AIDS, smoking and heart disease. The other reason, as Klein highlights, was money. The new emphasis on reducing demand by exercising control over GPs and the new stress on preventing illness were policies designed to manipulate the level of demand. Nor was this White Paper the end of journey by successive Conservative administrations back towards the public health paradigm.

In 1991 and 1992, the Major government produced Green and White Papers entitled *The health of the nation*. Klein sees this as a significant development in public policy, recognising that 'government had responsibilities for the health of the population that went beyond the provision of health services' (Klein, 1995: 210). Indeed, he argues that the roots of the strategy underlying these documents 'went back to the 19th century public health movement and the resurrection of this tradition internationally reflected the growing awareness that the role of medicine in producing health (as distinct from making the consequences of decay and disease more tolerable) was limited' (Klein, 1995: 210). It followed, therefore, that health was a cross-government responsibility and not merely one for the DH. Accordingly, a Cabinet Committee was established to coordinate policies and initiatives with potential impacts on health, and locally a series of 'healthy alliances' were proposed to promote locally integrated programmes focused on different sectors of public policy: healthy schools, healthy workplaces and healthy environments, for example. In addition, 25 national targets were set, for example, to reduce deaths from specific conditions such as heart disease and stroke, and to reduce the number of smokers and heavy drinkers. Although this approach undoubtedly represented a shift in thinking and contained aspects which were both consistent with Black and would not have been predicted from its dismissal by a previous Conservative administration, it fell well short of that Report's analysis and recommendations. Most particularly, it failed to acknowledge the impact of poverty and employment on health status. In addition, the combination of a Cabinet Committee, relatively undemanding targets and poorly articulated local 'healthy alliances' was an inadequate counterweight to the structural determinants of health identified by Black. As a result, this period of government is best seen as another stage in the re-emergence of public health but not one which saw a fundamental rebalancing between it and personal medicine. While recognising that the state and collectivist rather than purely individualist responses to health and premature mortality had legitimate roles, Klein's view that 'A Healthier Nation' marked a 'new health care paradigm' (1995: 211) seems overdrawn from the perspective developed here. Indeed, to describe it as a strategy for 'health care' is itself to point up its limitations in relation to the need to address underlying determinants of health.

Acheson Report, 1998

In the build-up to the 1997 general election the main focus of New Labour was on waiting lists and growth in financial resources available to the NHS (Sassi, 2005). However, before the election they announced the intention to have an independent inquiry into health inequalities as the first stage of long-term strategy to tackle the problem. On coming to power in 1997 the Labour government commissioned the Acheson Report, which was published in 1998, to review the latest available evidence on health inequalities, identify priority areas for future policy development and contribute to the development of a new strategy for health. The general conclusion of the Acheson Report was that 'for many aspects of health, inequality has generally worsened in the last few decades, especially in the 1980s and early 1990s' (Secretary of State for Health, 1999: para 4.5). Bambra et al note that:

> Acheson (1998) [like the Black Report] also supported a multi-causal approach to explaining health inequalities, using a model composed of different layers including individual lifestyles and the socioeconomic environment. Similarly to Black, this approach emphasised the importance of material and structural conditions in shaping other key determinants, such as lifestyle behaviours. (2011: 400)

Sassi (2005: 76–7) draws attention to three key elements of the Acheson report:

- the need for cross-governmental policies, at the national and local levels, to address the multidimensional causes of ill health;
- emphasis on a life-course approach – causes of health inequalities in adult life often date back to childhood / birth; and
- the need to address poverty and social exclusion as the primary objective of government policy, while recognising health inequalities tend to be shaped as a gradient across all social classes.

The report made 39 recommendations and Marmot, in his preface to *Tackling health inequalities: 2007 status report on the programme for action*, argues that 'importantly, Acheson took a social model of health. Thirty-six of its (our) recommendations ranged across the whole spectrum of government policy that influences health inequalities. Only three were specifically aimed at the health service' (DH, 2008: 5). Three of the recommendations were highlighted as particularly crucial and high priorities (Oliver, 2008; Bambra et al, 2011).

- All policies that are likely to have an impact on health should be evaluated in terms of their impact on health inequalities.
- A high priority should be given to the health of families with children, on the understanding that health in childhood can have a profound impact on all stages of the life course.
- Further steps should be taken to reduce income inequalities and improve the living standards of poor households.

In contrast to the Black Report, the Acheson Report was commissioned by a Labour government that had recently achieved a landslide victory, with a manifesto highlighting the need to tackle various social inequalities (Bambra et al, 2011). Sassi points out that the Report was generally warmly received, but 'seen as reflecting desirable goals more than concrete policy proposals' (2005: 77). In this respect, a key limitation of the Acheson Report was its failure to address explicitly trade-offs between equity and efficiency in relation to specific policies;

nor did it discuss how to prevent inequalities being worsened by other policies aimed at improving average health. Sassi (2005) contends that this would remain a crucial ambiguity in government policy.

New Labour's health inequalities policy

When Labour took office, most health indicators were showing long-term improvements but with a gradient in rates of improvement by socioeconomic condition, resulting in relentlessly increasing inequalities (Sassi, 2005: 71). In this respect, Graham (2004:116) highlights that England, like other older industrial countries, had seen a steady improvement in national health linked to increased national prosperity, but socioeconomic inequalities in risks (relative differences) of ill health and premature death remained and were matched by inequalities in the rates (absolute differences) of morbidity and mortality. The widening gap was deemed to reflect socioeconomic polarisation – widening gaps in income, income inequality, wealth and unemployment, and increasing rates of poverty in the most disadvantaged areas (Shaw et al, 1999; Graham, cited in Sassi, 2005).

Whitehead and Popay describe New Labour policies in England as providing 'perhaps the longest "natural policy experiment" in attempts to implement a purpose made action plan on health inequalities' (2010: 1235). Table 5.1 provides an overview of the development of this action plan, listing the major departmental publications around tackling health inequalities. On coming to office in 1997, the Labour government announced its aim (stemming from a dual concern with creating a fairer society and reducing the costs associated with ill health) to put health inequalities at the heart of tackling the root causes of ill health (NAO, 2010). However, progress in developing a strategy was relatively slow. Exworthy and Powell argue that 'it is notable that, even four years after its election and nearly three after the Acheson Inquiry report was published, the government launched in 2001 a consultation on a "plan for delivery" of policies tackling health inequalities, drawing on the views of local stakeholders' (2004: 271). While this ultimately led to *Tackling health inequalities: A programme for action* (DH, 2003) and subsequent related policy documents and progress reports, it also draws attention to the difficulty the government had in devising a comprehensive strategy for this issue. Moreover, devising the strategy formed only part of the task: agreeing its priority within the wider programme of government was also significant issue. Despite publishing a public service agreement (PSA) target around health inequalities in 2002, the National Audit Office (NAO) notes that 'it took until 2006, more than three years from the publication of the health inequalities strategy and half way through the lifetime of the PSA target, for the Department to establish health inequalities as a top six NHS priority' (NAO, 2010: 12).

Table 5.1: Tackling health inequalities – major departmental publications

Year	Title	Description
1998	*Independent inquiry into inequalities in health report*	Independent review of health inequalities by Sir Donald Acheson
2000	*The NHS Plan*	Announced the creation of a specific PSA target to reduce health inequalities, officially announced in February 2001
2002	*Tackling health inequalities: A cross-cutting review*	Department of Health/HM Treasury joint review to establish priorities for future action to address health inequalities
2003	*Tackling health inequalities: A programme for action*	A response to the cross-cutting review, which established 82 indicators for improvement across 12 departments by 2006
2004	*HM Treasury spending review 2004*	Health inequalities PSA target retained but amended to measure the gap between England and Spearhead local authorities from April 2005
2005	*Tackling health inequalities: what works*	Current thinking on cost-effective interventions to reduce health inequalities
2006	*NHS operating framework 2006–07*	Health inequalities named as one of the NHS' top six priorities
2008	*Tackling health inequalities: Status report on the programme for action*	Update on progress against the PSA target
2008	*Tackling health inequalities: Progress and next steps*	Actions to re-focus attention on achieving the 2010 target in the wake of the completion of the programme for action
2008	*Systematically addressing health inequalities*	Good practice identified from early visits by the National Support Team for Health Inequalities
2008	*Tackling health inequalities: 2005–07 policy and data update for the 2010 national target*	Update on progress against the PSA target
2009	*Government response to the Health Select Committee report on health inequalities*	Government's statement of actions across departments that address parliamentary findings and recommendations about work to tackle health inequalities

Source: NAO (2010: 45)

The Green Paper *Our healthier nation* (Secretary of State for Health, 1998) and the White Paper *Saving lives* (Secretary of State for Health, 1999) promised to deliver more accessible and continuously improving services, while also focusing on ill health and inequalities. The *Saving lives* White Paper indicates that individual behaviour is often vital to health, but stresses that 'poor health can spring from a complex interaction between the genetic makeup and behaviour of individuals and social, economic and environmental factors in the community' (Secretary of State for Health, 1999: para 1.4). Consequently, the government adopted an approach targeted on working across government to 'attack the breeding ground for poor health – poverty and social exclusion' (Secretary of State for Health, 1999: para 1.7). In this respect, the structural determinants of health, highlighted by Acheson, formed a key strand of New Labour's policy from the outset. However, Dorling (2013b) notes that in practice the government failed to prioritise the fundamental drivers of social inequality beyond changes in social and fiscal policy, which cannot be expected to eradicate such inequalities. He cites Hills et al and Goldthorpe to claim that surprisingly little was done to alter the fundamental structure of social inequalities in the UK. This is borne out by the level of income inequality in the UK, which has remained consistently high since the neoliberal reforms of the Thatcher governments of the 1980s (this is discussed more fully in Chapter Two in the section on inequality).

Nevertheless, this theme remained a prominent strand in the New Labour government's health inequalities rhetoric and was developed further in the subsequent cross–cutting review on health inequalities:

> Health inequalities follow a social gradient, with the health gap increasing steadily with poorer social class. Because of this gradient, and the distribution of the population in the different social groups, analysis shows that interventions must reach more than the most deprived areas and the most disadvantaged/socially excluded populations to meet the national targets and make progress on health inequalities more generally. (DH, 2002: 2)

Tackling health inequalities: A cross-cutting review also refined the government's earlier target (from the 2000 spending review) to 'narrow the gap between socio-economic groups and between the most deprived areas and the rest of the country, in childhood and throughout life' (NAO, 2010: 5). The new target took the form of a PSA and was concerned with reducing inequalities by 2010 in health outcomes by 10% as measured by infant mortality and life expectancy at birth (DH, 2002). At this time the government also turned its attention to population-wide health measures such as the ban on direct and indirect promotion or advertising of tobacco products through the Tobacco Advertising and Promotion Act 2002. This was followed by regulations to enforce a smoking ban in public areas under part one of the Health Act 2006. In addition, campaigns around healthy eating (such as those concerning five fruit and vegetables a day and childhood obesity) emerged in the mid- to late-2000s (Buck and Frosini, 2012) as part of this drive towards introducing population-wide health measures. However, Buck and Frosini also contend that 'although recognised as important in reducing inequality in the long run, the changing of unhealthy behaviours was not a priority in the drive by the Department of Health to meet its target on life expectancy gaps agreed with the Prime Minister's Delivery Unit' (2012: 14).

Returning to the health inequalities agenda, much of the government's early work around health inequalities led to the DH producing *Tackling health inequalities: A programme for action* (2003). The document set out plans to tackle health inequalities in the short term, and established the foundations to achieve the national PSA target. The NAO states that the strategy 'called on PCTs [primary care trusts] and strategic health authorities to ensure that tackling health inequalities was central to their planning and performance systems. It included 12 cross-government headline indicators and 82 cross-government commitments' (2010: 5). However, the NAO (2010) points out that the 2003 health inequalities strategy lacked effective mechanisms to drive delivery against the target. It attributes this to the knowledge base for health inequalities at this time still being under construction. The 2004 Wanless report on *Securing good health for the whole population* also argues that the programme for action gave no indication of how much various aspects of the strategy would contribute towards meeting the health inequality targets, and that as a result it would be difficult to prioritise action at a local level. The *Choosing health* White Paper went some way towards addressing issues around prioritising action by setting 'out action to address inequalities in health that focuses particularly on getting information across to people in different groups and securing better access to healthier choices for people in disadvantaged groups or areas' (DH, 2004b: 6). Meanwhile, some of the issues around the knowledge base were addressed through *Tackling health inequalities: What works* (DH, 2005), which identified interventions for health priority areas.

In the 2004 Treasury spending review, the PSA target was reaffirmed and underpinned by two more detailed objectives:

- starting with children under one year, by 2010 to reduce by at least 10 per cent the gap in mortality between the routine and manual group and the population as a whole;
- starting with local authorities, by 2010 to reduce by at least 10 per cent the gap in life expectancy between the fifth of areas with the worst health and deprivation indicators (the Spearhead Group) and the population as a whole. (HM Treasury, 2004: 13)

Consequently, since 2004 action to tackle health inequalities was increasingly focused on the Spearhead group of local authority areas, which were expected to make faster progress in meeting the national health inequality targets. The Spearhead group consisted of the 70 local authority areas, which mapped onto 62 PCTs that were in the bottom fifth nationally for three or more of the following five factors:

- male life expectancy at birth;
- female life expectancy at birth;
- cancer mortality rate in under–75s;
- cardiovascular disease mortality rate in under–75s; and
- Index of Multiple Deprivation 2004 (Local Authority Summary), average score (DH, 2007a: 3).

While the Spearhead areas represented the local authority areas with the worst health and deprivation, considerable 'pockets' of deprivation and poor health were concentrated outside the Spearhead group. In fact, the NAO (2010) highlights that under half (48%) of local authority wards with the worst life expectancy were in Spearhead areas.

By the middle of the 2000s it was becoming clear that there were wide variations across PCT areas in England in making progress towards the government's 2010 national health inequality targets (DH, 2006; 2007a). All the Spearhead PCTs were issued with trajectories in all-age–all-cause mortality necessary for them to meet the 2010 targets, with the expectation that they would plan their interventions to meet these trajectories. The implications of the trajectories and the original 2010 endpoint is that interventions exist which, individually or in combination, can be shown to be capable of delivering the specified change over the specified period. Whether such evidence underpinned the target setting process is not clear but seems unlikely. For example, there was little evidence about what might be behind the differential performance of Spearhead areas because no systematic research was undertaken to compare each area as a 'case'. It was not clear, for example, whether the Spearheads missing the targets were slow to build capacity in smoking cessation clinics, whether their primary care organisations had been reactive rather than proactive with secondary prevention, or whether other factors to do with ways of working, leadership or local context were behind these differences. A study that adopted just such an approach, together with the findings from it, is the subject of Chapter Eight.

The NAO (2010) notes that from 2006 to 2007 a series of measures was introduced to promote action to address health inequalities, including the following.

- Health inequalities became a top six NHS priority in 2006, alongside the requirement for PCTs to report on action taken. PCTs were reorganised to more closely align with local authority boundaries.Strategic health authorities increased monitoring of the inequality gap in all-age-all-cause mortality indicator.NHS and local government performance-management systems were aligned through the use of the all-age-all-cause mortality indicator in both systems.The Health Inequalities National Support Team was established in 2007 to provide support to local areas, focusing principally on the life expectancy element of the 2010 PSA target.
- The health inequalities intervention tool was made available to help PCTs and local authorities.

The limited progress made towards meeting the health inequalities targets (DH, 2008) triggered the setting up of the Marmot Review in 2008 (Whitehead and Popay, 2010). The political climate was quite different from the time the Acheson Report was commissioned, as the government was not enjoying public or media support at this time (Bambra et al, 2011). The government had also moved away from its early commitment to tackling 'upstream' structural determinants of health and was more focused on 'downstream' individual lifestyle factors (Bambra et al, 2011). We will turn to the recommendations of the Marmot Review and the implications of these for the Coalition government's policy in relation to health inequalities in the next chapter (in the section on austerity). In addition, Chapter Six begins with an overview of New Labour's record in terms of health inequality outcomes, which provides useful context to the Coalition's agenda in this area by outlining the nature and extent of health inequalities today.

Conclusion

This chapter has focused on the development of public policy towards the improvement of health outcomes and the reduction of inequalities in health status. It has sought to understand these issues through the lenses provided by the public health and personal medicine paradigms for intervening to prevent disease and restore health. From this perspective, we have shown that the earliest state interventions were based on the former approach but the establishment of the NHS was essentially shaped by the latter. Although there has been renewed interest in the public health paradigm in recent years, the personal medicine paradigm continues to underpin the principal 'common sense' understanding of public policy interventions to improve health. At the same time, however, understandings of the limitations of this approach have begun to influence the direction of policy development. Such understandings are associated with three different but not unrelated challenges to the role of personal medical services: first, that they had been less important historically than public health interventions in reducing premature mortality; second, that the evidence base for much clinical practice was lacking; and third, that not only could medicine produce positively harmful outcomes but also medical imperialism had so captured the terms of debate that socioeconomic determinants of health, along with strategies to ameliorate them, received insufficient attention.

These limitations help us to understand the persistence of inequalities in health outcomes alongside the existence of universal and comprehensive health services free at the point of delivery. In practice, the NHS was a vehicle for universalising personal medical services but not for eradicating (or even seeking to eradicate) inequalities in health and life expectancy. The most it could hope to achieve was to eradicate financial barriers to access and secure universal access based on need to a consistent range and quality of services across the population as a whole. In the first half of the twentieth century these were necessary goals, and their pursuit continues to be a critical contribution to securing equality of access to treatment and care according to need rather than income, geography or social position.

What the NHS could not do was seriously challenge, and still less eradicate, inequalities in health derived from the influence of socioeconomic factors determining morbidity and mortality because, on its own, the underlying operating model of personal medicine is not fit for that purpose. From this perspective, the most fundamental limitation of the personal medical paradigm is the extent to which it has come to be seen as a near universal model for addressing what is in reality a set of wicked problems. As a result, public policy has tended to conflate and oversimplify the related, but quite different, issues of promoting universal access to health services, restoring health cost-effectively and reducing inequalities in healthy life expectancy. In so doing, the logic model adopted for understanding and addressing health inequalities has been too readily restricted to one which mirrors the medical model's concern to treat symptoms more than causes, and gives too little attention to the interplay between individual agency and the underlying structural determinants of health.

SIX

Health inequalities post 2010

Introduction

> Health inequalities have ceased to be fashionable. From a
> position where the goal to reduce inequalities was a core
> objective of the health system – with national targets to
> reduce them by 10 per cent – we have seen it steadily
> marginalised. In a few short years the goal of social equality
> in health has been reduced to trying, not very hard, to
> ensure decent access to health care for those in the most
> disadvantaged groups. (Scally, 2013)

Gregory et al (2012) point out that the Coalition government accepted
most of the recommendations of the Marmot Review, with the
exception of the prescription to narrow income inequalities. This is
a significant exception and one that separates an apparent concern
with intervening to reduce health inequalities from some of the core
structural inequalities in society. However, the extent to which this is
a significant departure from New Labour's approach to tackling health
inequalities is open to debate. In practice, it can be argued that the latter
was primarily characterised by a focus on equality of opportunities,
rather than challenging structurally located socioeconomic sources of
inequality, and on policies aimed at reducing poverty (among children
in particular) that at best stemmed, but did not reverse, the trend in
rising inequalities (see Sefton and Sutherland, 2005, for a much fuller
discussion). Consequently, this apparently significant cleavage could be
regarded as consistent with a much longer trend of official responses
to health inequalities falling short (Glasby, 2012).

This chapter focuses mainly on the Coalition government and on its
policies for improving health and reducing health inequalities. Before
we develop that analysis, however, we examine evidence about the
New Labour legacy in terms of its record on health inequalities and its
impact on the social gradient in health. This is followed by a discussion
of the programme of austerity that frames much of the Coalition
government's agenda and policies. We then move on to focus on a
key narrative shaping the Coalition's approach to governance: the 'Big

Society'. The next section then outlines a number of key features of the Coalition's health policies and the chapter concludes with a discussion of the potential implications of those policies for health inequalities.

New Labour's record on health inequalities

> The persistence of inequalities in population health outcomes was highlighted at the beginning of Labour's period in power in the Acheson Report (1998) and at the end of Labour's period in power in the Marmot Review (2010). (Vizard and Obolenskaya, 2013: 95)

The context for New Labour's record in tackling health inequalities is provided by the relationship between its spending priorities and the social determinants of health outlined in Chapter One in the section on potential causes, together with outcomes associated with such expenditures. Our principal sources for reviewing the impact of these spending programmes are two recently published audits of New Labour's period in office by the Centre for Analysis of Social Exclusion. In the first, Lupton et al (2013) argue that the New Labour government set out to deliver ambitious social goals, a starting point which marked a radical change in direction from the previous Conservative government. They assert that:

> While seemingly ambivalent about overall inequality and in particular the position of the very rich, Labour made explicit commitments to tackling poverty and social exclusion, tackling inequalities in health and educational outcomes, and to improving neighbourhood conditions and life chances for those in the poorest areas. (2013: 60)

Overall inequality is an important factor in relation to these outcomes, and not challenging the structure of the economy or society and the inequalities within them arguably undermined the more progressive aims of New Labour's social policy. Poverty, social exclusion, education and health outcomes are all, to some degree, relative concepts. How a child performs in school or how healthy someone is throughout their life course is associated with (but not, at an individual level, wholly determined by) socioeconomic contextual variables and their differential impact on individuals, groups and places. At an aggregate level the relationship between health outcomes and socioeconomic variables has been well demonstrated by, for example, Black (1980) and

Marmot (2010). Inequality clearly matters to health status, therefore, but, as we argued in Chapter One, so too does the extent to which policy recognises, and is capable of challenging, the social and economic determinants of health. Thus, the impact of initiatives to reduce health inequalities is dependent on, first, the extent to which the state is seen to have a role in modifying the inequalities that are (re)produced across society; and, second, in the extent its governance structures enable it to identify and address social determinants in health effectively.

One interpretation of New Labour's programme in government was that it did not seek (and arguably missed an opportunity) to restore a socioeconomic and governance model based on more collectivist social norms, but instead grafted elements of social support and social investment onto neoliberal policies (Coates, 2010). However, Grimshaw and Rubery (2012) contend that the neoliberal approach to economic organisation and desire to control inflation was exploited by New Labour to create space for increases in public spending amounting to an average annual growth rate of 3.2% between 1997/8 and 2007/8, compared with 1.5% between 1979/80 and 1996/7. Lupton et al (2013) highlight that the expansion of public spending under New Labour went towards reinvestment in, and 'modernisation' of, public services to bring the UK more in line with other European countries following the period of comparatively low spending under the previous Conservative government. During New Labour's period of office public spending increased from £449 billion in 1996/7 to £725 billion in 2009/10 (a rise of 60%). This spending growth occurred during a period where GDP (Gross Domestic Product) increased by 30%; it represented an increase in public spending as a proportion of GDP from 39.5% to 47.4% (Lupton et al, 2013). Over the same period health spending increased from 5.3% of GDP to 8.3%, which was more than twice the rate of the overall increase in public spending (Lupton et al, 2013). The impact on health inequalities of such increases in public spending overall or on the National Health Service (NHS) more specifically is another matter, but Lupton et al (2013: 60) show that increased public expenditure reduced but did not eliminate socioeconomic variations in access to services.

However, investment in and access to services is just one element in a comprehensive strategy to reduce health inequalities. As we argued in the previous chapter, spending on the provision of health services, though not unimportant, is essentially a response to the symptoms and not the causes of illness and disability. To the extent that those underlying causes are rooted in social and economic inequalities, spending on health services, even to reduce inequalities of access, can have only a limited impact on inequalities of health outcomes between socioeconomic groups and classes. The National Audit Office (NAO) review of New Labour initiatives to reduce health inequalities identifies three categories of causes of health inequalities: wider determinants (such as financial status and housing); the lives people lead (including risk factors such as alcohol, tobacco and obesity); and the health services people use (together with the accessibility and responsiveness of all of these) (2010: 4). Clearly, services have a role to play in each of these areas but the 'complex mix of social, economic, cultural and political reasons' highlighted by the NAO (2010: 4) also relates more fundamentally to the socioeconomic organisation and structure of society and how resources are distributed within it.

Lupton et al's review of policy, spending and outcomes during the New Labour period concludes that:

> there remained a long way still go towards a more equal society after all the spending. Overall income inequality fell slightly as a result of the crash but had not been falling before that and remained high by international standards, as did overall relative poverty rates. Large socio-economic gaps remained on most indicators. International data on the change in the UK's international position are disappointing for health and inconclusive for education. One conclusion from this could be that 'spending doesn't work'. However this is not supported either at the general or specific level. In general terms, where Labour spent money, outcomes shifted, while on areas on which no policy effort or extra money was expended, outcomes remained unchanged. Specific research tended to show that more spending was better than less spending, although there were questions about value for money of certain policies. Another conclusion is that socio-economic inequalities in outcomes are hard to shift, in the context of persistent high inequality – that there are limits to what social policies can achieve in the absence of economic change. (2013: 61)

The last comment is of particular relevance to our analysis here of the underlying socioeconomic determinants of health and the limited impact of health services on their amelioration. The 56% increase in spending on the NHS by the Blair and Brown administrations, compared with 20% growth in overall public expenditure (Lupton et al, 2013), was primarily focused on enabling more people to access health services more quickly (Appleby et al, 2010) through the various waiting-time initiatives. As the end of New Labour's period in office approached, the NAO (2010) reported that only about 2% of primary care trust (PCT) spending was in the category of preventing illness and promoting good health, including smoking cessation services. One conclusion to be drawn from these comparisons is that, in terms of national priorities, spending on health services was favoured over that on other services, especially local government, which might have been targeted on some of the underlying causes of health inequalities (though inequalities of income are a separate issue, as we suggest below). Furthermore, this increased spending tended to reinforce the imbalance between personal medicine and initiatives to target the social and economic determinants of health and health inequalities. Turner et al provide a further example, noting that 'PCTs have struggled to get large provider trusts and general practitioners [GPs] to look beyond the patients they see and take responsibility for tackling inequalities in the health of the wider population' (2013: 2). The introduction of the Quality and Outcomes Framework (QOF) in 2003, for example, led to GP practices being financially rewarded for meeting specific clinical activity targets. However, the NAO (2010) and Dixon et al (2011) state that the impact of the QOF on health inequalities has been limited as these QOF do not focus sufficiently on the neediest groups and many of these targets can be met without tackling health inequalities and by excluding 'difficult' cases, providing little incentive for practices to undertake primary prevention or public health interventions.[32]

A further, and arguably more fundamental, criticism of New Labour's approach to tackling health inequalities has focused on its unwillingness to move very far from the neoliberal[33] governance agenda established by the previous Conservative government, with its acceptance of higher levels of income inequality as an engine of growth in a globalised economy. In practice, the evidence is mixed. Improvements in economic prosperity were secured but not shared equally, with employment and incomes improving at slower rates in some regions than others (Barr et al, 2012), and particularly in those where health inequalities were most pronounced. In that respect, economic policy can be seen to have reinforced rather than challenged socioeconomic determinants of health. Nevertheless, Lupton et al (2013) conclude that some social and economic outcomes improved, especially for those groups explicitly targeted by policy – such as pensioners and families with children. They anticipate that the increased spending on education and early years is likely to have continued benefits into adulthood. Finally, they show that while income inequality fell slightly, it did so only due to economic depression[34] and remains high by international standards.

As explained in Chapters One and Five, the English public service agreement (PSA) targets related to reductions in health inequalities had two main strands:

- **infant mortality** – a target to reduce by 10% in 2010, the gap in mortality for children under one year old between the 'routine and manual occupation group' and the population as a whole;
- **life expectancy** – a target to reduce by at least 10% in 2010 the gap between the fifth of areas with the worst health and deprivation indicators (the 'Spearhead' group of local authorities) and the population as a whole.

Vizard and Obolenskaya (2013), in the second report from the Centre of Analysis of Social Exclusion mentioned above, argue that despite initially slow progress it appears that the infant mortality target will have been met (with one year of data outstanding), as the most recent figures suggests that the absolute[35] and relative[36] gaps fell by 42% and 25% respectively over the period 1997/9 to 2008/10. While this is undoubtedly a success in terms of the policy goals set by the New Labour government, it is important to recognise that the second PSA target is of wider significance in terms of its impact on the health of the population overall. As we have already argued, what really matters in terms of health inequalities is whether we have a decent quality of life and acceptable life span before we die. In this respect, and despite an increase in life expectancy for men by 3.8 years and women by 2.6 years between 1995/7 and 2008/10 in the Spearhead areas (where health inequalities were greatest), the improvements in health lagged behind the all–England rate and, consequently, inequality increased. The relative gaps increased for both men and women during this period from 2.57% to 2.61% and 1.77% to 2.00% respectively, which implies that the life expectancy inequality target is not expected to be met (although a final verdict will require the 2009/11 data). Moreover, while people are living longer, the proportion of their lives spent disability-free is decreasing marginally and there has been a modest increase in the gap between the least deprived fifth of areas, where people can expect to live 85% of their lives disability-free compared with 74% for those living in the most deprived areas (Vizard and Obolenskaya, 2013).

According to Vizard and Obolenskaya, the 2004 cancers PSA target to reduce the absolute gap in inequalities by at least 6% between the

Spearhead areas and the population as a whole is likely to be met (although a final evaluation for 2009/11 is required). The absolute gap between England and the Spearhead areas was 20.7 deaths per 100,000 population in 1995/7, reducing to 18.3 by 2008/10. This represented an 11.6% narrowing of the absolute gap, although the relative gap grew by 13.4% in the same period (2013: 102–3).[37] The 2004 PSA target for circulatory diseases aimed at a 40% reduction in the absolute inequalities gap between the Spearhead areas and the population as a whole. Vizard and Obolenskaya (2013) state that there was an 'impressive' 50.9% fall in the death rate in Spearhead areas, but that this rate of improvement lagged behind the all-England average of a 52.4% fall in the death rate. Consequently, the relative gap increased in the period 1995/97 to 2008/10. However, the absolute gap did fall by 45.2% in the same period, suggesting that the target will be met, with one year's data still outstanding. These apparent achievements do, however, need to be viewed in the light of the NAO (2010) argument that the cancers and circulatory disease targets were set too low to make a significant contribution to meeting the overall life expectancy target. Furthermore, the NAO (2010) identifies a number of challenges for New Labour's health inequalities strategy that include the lack of a knowledge base around the cost–effectiveness and overall effectiveness of measures to tackle health inequalities and insufficient prioritisation (until it became a top six NHS priority in 2006) in policy and planning. Somewhat similarly, Turner et al (2013: 2) outline four persistent lines of critique for the disappointing progress towards health inequality targets:

- lack of attention to social and economic inequality;
- failure to shift resources from secondary and tertiary care to high-quality prevention, early diagnosis and treatment in primary care;lack of performance management; and
- persistence of weak evidence base.

The above discussion suggests there are at least two somewhat different ways to view New Labour's record on health inequalities. The first relates to the impact of wider macroeconomic policies and New Labour's apparently enthusiastic adoption of a neoliberal economic model. In this respect, Pearce states that:

> the unequal distribution of social factors, including employment, education, and housing, have been underpinned in many countries including the UK by the rapid implementation of market oriented economic and

social policies over the past three decades which have been designed to deregulate the labour market and constrain social security. (2013: 2033)

To this we would add the unequal distribution of health (as Pearce does in his article), and how this is a product of these market-oriented policies. The second way of viewing New Labour's record is outlined by Grimshaw and Rubery (2012) and relates to the repeated and consistent attempts to 'square the circle of neo-liberalism with a human face' through the investment in services outlined above. Both these views have some merit but the former is, arguably, more persuasive in explaining the persistence of underlying causes of health inequalities, given the continued significance of the social gradient in health. In view of this pattern of outcomes from the New Labour administrations, prospects for reducing health inequalities look even more testing in the current climate of austerity. As Lupton et al suggest, 'given the relatively modest progress towards greater social justice that could be made over 13 years of consistent policy effort at high spending levels, making greater strides in the current financial situation must be seen as a tough challenge' (2013: 62). We consider the implications of this conclusion below.

Austerity

The 2008 financial crisis had its origins in the banking sector but its consequences have been profound in other sectors and for public services in particular (Crouch, 2011). The British economy was especially hard hit by the crisis due to the (over)reliance on financial services following the deindustrialisation of the economy (Doetter and Gotze, 2011).[38] Despite political claims that 'we are all in this together', there remain continuing concerns (see, for example, Barr et al, 2012; Clarke and Newman, 2012; Pearce, 2013) that the impacts of this crisis will not be evenly shared, with some sections of the population hit harder than others. Pearce (2013) and Barr et al (2012) specifically highlight health and wellbeing as an area likely to be negatively affected by the crisis and subsequent austerity measures, as we discuss below.

The Conservative/Liberal Democrat Coalition government which succeeded New Labour in 2010 adopted a programme of fiscal austerity as a necessary response, it argued, to a budget deficit and total public sector net debt at levels higher than at any time since 1975. Combined with the consequential borrowing requirements were growing pressures of demand on public spending from population ageing and a rising birth rate (Lupton et al, 2013). The new government's central priority, as outlined in the Coalition Agreement, was to balance the budget by the end of the 2014/15 financial year: 'the deficit reduction programme takes precedence over any of the other measures in this agreement' (Cabinet Office, 2010a). Porter points out that in reducing the deficit 'the emphasis thus far has been on driving down public spending rather than increasing progressive tax income. Thus, the brunt of austerity has been taken by those who are either employed by the state or who depend on state services' (2013: 7). In practice, borrowing has remained significantly higher than originally planned and the date for bringing state finances into balance has been pushed back, with very substantial spending reductions programmed into 2018 (IFS, 2014). However, the implications identified by Porter hold true.

The Coalition government sought to cut the spending deficit from 8.4% of GDP in 2009 to 0.4% in 2015, and to reverse the growth of public debt in four years, rather than the 14 recommended by the OECD (Taylor-Gooby, 2012). The spending review of October 2010 brought the total value of cuts to £81 billion, aiming to eliminate the structural deficit by 2015, although this was subsequently revised to 2018. The public sector workforce was to be cut by 490,000 jobs, with an average departmental budget cut of 19% over four years and a further £7 billion cut from the welfare budget (Lowndes and Pratchett, 2012). Those regions and localities that have a larger proportion of public sector workers are likely to be hardest hit by these austerity measures. Indeed, Office for National Statistics (ONS) data (cited in Pearce, 2013) indicates that between 2008 and 2012 all regions in England[39] have seen a reduction in the public sector workforce, but this varies between 12% in the North East and 3.4% in the South East.

It is also important to recognise that the spending cuts are not being targeted equally across different parts of the public sector. In fact, the Coalition made a commitment to increase health spending in real terms in every year of the parliament (DH, 2010b). As Professor Tony Travers argued in his evidence to the Public Accounts Committee:

> if you look at the period from 2010–11, the base year for the spending review, through to 2014–15, then, as predicted, local government spending, on average, will have fallen by 14%. The equivalent number for the NHS is plus 12.3%, so one is going one way and the other is going the other way. (Public Accounts Committee, 2013: Q57)

When education, police and fire are excluded from the analysis, the 2010 spending review plans for reductions in central government's funding to local authorities are even more pronounced, and amount to a reduction of 26% in real terms over four years. Consequently, local authorities are bearing a higher proportion of public spending reductions than other sectors (Lowndes and Pratchett, 2012). Given the significance of the social determinants of health for health inequalities and the role of non-NHS providers in tackling these, there are real grounds for concern about the likely impact of current spending programmes on health inequalities. Such concerns are underpinned by the NAO's recommendation that 'the DH [Department of Health] and NHS cannot tackle health inequalities without strong partnership working across government' (2010: 13), which they relate to DH estimates that around only 15–20% of inequalities in mortality rates can be directly influenced by health interventions which prevent or reduce the risk of ill health.

The partnerships the NAO refers to include substantial roles for local government, given its responsibilities for a wide range of social and environmental services[40] but, as we have noted above, central government grant funding to local authorities was to be cut by over a quarter in real terms (£7.6 billion) between 2011 and 2015 (Public Accounts Committee, 2013: 3). The nature of local funding is also set to change from one in which all business rates revenue was pooled nationally and redistributed to local authorities according to a formula designed to reflect relative needs and ability to raise income tax locally. However, from 2013/14, local authorities will retain approximately 50% of business rates raised locally (Public Accounts Committee, 2013: 7). The intention was to incentivise the promotion of local business growth but, in the short term at least, the implications for health inequalities are potentially concerning. The areas with more need may have less scope to raise local business revenue, given that these tend to be the areas that have coped less well with the economic consequences of deindustrialisation and subsequent shifts to a more service-based economy.

More generally, the Department for Communities and Local Government (DCLG) itself accepts that it is inevitable that the local authorities that are more grant-dependent will be harder hit by government reductions in funding. Indeed, the Public Accounts Committee notes that 'so far the highest reductions in terms of spending power have tended to be for councils that depend most on government grants, where needs for local services tend to be greatest' (2013: 3), with the levels of reduction in individual authorities varying from just over 1% to nearly 9% in 2012/13. Pearce (2013) has calculated the mean reduction in spending power for all English local authorities between 2012/13 and 2013/14 and stratified this into deprivation quintiles (using the 2010 English Indices of Deprivation). He reveals a linear trend here of spending power declining as deprivation levels increase, with the result that reductions in spending are consistently higher in the most socially disadvantaged local authorities. Clarke and Newman assert that 'this points to the ways in which new landscapes of inequality get mapped on to existing ones, since both public service use and benefits are already (largely) "targeted" on vulnerable and impoverished groups' (2012: 306). This pattern has important implications for the social gradient in health. For example, Pearce argues that many of the austerity measures risk affecting the social determinants of health and exacerbating health inequalities, because these are 'affected by complex and long-term processes that reflect socially patterned exposures in early life and the cumulative effect of experiences in later life' (2013: 2033).

Pearce (2013) similarly points out that not only will the availability and quality of key services be compromised, so will employment levels, job security, infrastructure and income equality, all of which are causally related to health status. We are also likely to see heightened regional disparities in health status resulting from growing spatial concentrations of inequalities. This is significant because the degree to which inequalities are concentrated spatially and among particular groups has been found to be associated with healthy behaviours and their improvement. For example, Buck and Frosini found that while the clustering of unhealthy behaviours has been in decline in England in recent years, the decline is primarily concentrated in higher socioeconomic and educational groups. They contend that more broadly based change in behaviours will require holistic approaches to policy and practice that help people in lower socioeconomic groups to change their lifestyles and reduce unhealthy behaviours (Buck and Frosini, 2012). However, there are significant inconsistencies between the demands of such holistic approaches and current policies for the economy and public expenditure. Indeed, Grimshaw and Rubery claim that the continuation of 'the neoliberal agenda with a shrinking rather than growing state is likely to see a weakened responsiveness to social needs' (2012: 118).

There are also concerns about the extent to which consequences of the austerity programme have been thought through. For example, the Public Accounts Committee concludes that the DCLG 'did not do enough work with other departments to model how funding changes may adversely affect other areas of the public sector, for example cuts in local authority adult social care could lead to bed blocking in hospitals'. Furthermore, 'the Department [DCLG] needs to work with other departments to improve central government's assessment of the effects of funding reductions and reforms – including how they interact with each other – before the next spending review' (Public Accounts Committee, 2013: 3, 5). Similarly, a study by the Nuffield Trust and Health Foundation (Ismail et al, 2014: 7) suggests that cuts in publicly funded adult social care services were very likely to be having negative consequences for older people's health and wellbeing and that of their carers, but poor linkage between health and social care data at a national level means that it is currently difficult to quantify the impact.

The Public Accounts Committee's (2013) conclusion that DCLG does not really understand the impact of spending reductions and funding changes on individual councils and poorer or more vulnerable communities demonstrates that the consequences of austerity are yet to be fully identified and understood. However, as Pearce (2013) argues, it seems clear that austerity measures are not going to be shared equally across the country; socially and economically disadvantaged areas which tend to have poorer health outcomes are likely to be more affected than other areas. Allen (2013) agrees, emphasising that health inequalities continue to widen across England and that the Institute of Health Equity's analysis suggests that this progress has been exacerbated both by the economic circumstances since 2008 and by more recent Coalition reforms to welfare benefits. She concludes that this combination of recession and austerity is likely to widen health inequalities considerably.

Big Society

In Chapter Two (in the section on complexity) we discussed the significance of 'place' and health outcomes. In England there has been a growing focus on neighbourhoods and communities through a trend towards 'localism'[41] in policy (Castelli et al, 2013: 3). The development of the Big Society narrative by the Conservatives prior to the 2010 election and subsequently adopted by the Coalition government can be seen as the most recent iteration of this trend. Dawson summarises the main concern for Big Society advocates as the growth and pervasiveness of the state, which 'is seen to: create dependence; stifle localised, and thus specialised, forms of organisation; lessen individual liberty; and destroy subsidiarity (moral responsibility for the local)' (2013: 88). While the rhetoric around the Big Society declined as the Coalition government's term in office progressed, the concern with the growth of the state has remained an underlying philosophy cutting across the Coalition programme. This, in turn, has led to a new focus on localism and communities that is arguably of potentially great significance for health inequalities, and forms much of the discussion in this section.

The Coalition Agreement defined three core components of the Big Society agenda as:

- empowering communities – giving local councils and neighbourhoods more power to take decisions and shape their area;
- opening up public services – enabling charities, social enterprises, private companies and employee-owned cooperatives to compete to offer people high quality services; and
- promoting social action – encouraging and enabling people from all walks of life to play a more active part in society, and promoting more volunteering and philanthropy (Cabinet Office, 2010b: 3).

Buser describes the Big Society thus:

> Framed by a programme of public spending cuts and fiscal austerity, these reforms do more than alter the scale of public service; they present a re-conceptualisation of citizen engagement in which individuals, the private sector, and third sector groups are set to gain a variety of responsibilities for the management of civic space and the provision of public services. (2013: 3)

He continues by noting that in the Big Society rhetoric there is a distinct notion of democracy, where civic engagement and participation act as precursors to democratic renewal and mending 'our broken society' (2013: 7). Through the Big Society the state has a role in fixing 'broken Britain' through moral suasion and by distributing and giving power away to citizens, but does not have a role in addressing economic and social inequalities (Lakin, 2013). The Coalition government's 'broken society' narrative focuses on a perceived social and moral decay linked to a variety of 'problem' behaviours in socially disadvantaged (and highly stigmatised) neighbourhoods (Pearce, 2013). This rhetoric about the erosion of moral standards is strongly linked to dependency on the welfare state among some groups of people (Hancock and Mooney, 2013). However, according to Dawson, it does so by overlooking economic inequality, and 'by tying political devolution to continued economic deregulation, it is more likely to increase and retrench current forms of inequality and fragmentation' (2013: 79).

The lack of attention to the stratification of society is an important feature of the Big Society concept and shares similarities with Charles Murray's frequently criticised conception of the underclass (see Murray, 1984, for example). Murray's work was regarded by many (see Wilson, 1987; Byrne, 2005, for example) as essentially 'bad social science' and a largely *culturalist* explanation. The Big Society's focus on 'broken Britain' is very similar because it pays little attention to the implications of the types of power inequalities generated by social and economic inequalities in society (see, for example, Glasman, 2010; ACEVO, 2011; Dorling, 2011; 2013b; Corbett and Walker, 2013). Consequently, much of the case for the Big Society is based on individualist and culturalist explanations, emphasising agency but neglecting the implications of structural factors for individuals' actions. Essentially, we need to go one step further back than the Big Society narrative about broken Britain goes. Put simply, if something is broken what has broken it? It can be argued (and has been in the Big Society narrative) that it is dependency on the state that has done so, but we must also ask what has created such dependency. Byrne (2005) points out that the ideology of liberal capitalism in post-Fordist and post-industrial societies is creating social policies organised around flexible labour markets and structural exclusion. In this respect, the UK moved from a post-war period of near full unemployment to an unemployment rate that has rarely fallen below 5% (on occasions reaching over 10%) from the 1980s onwards (ONS, 2014b June Labour Market statistics). At the time of writing the unemployment rate is falling but doing so against a near doubling of the part-time employment rate since 2008 (ONS, 2013a) and a lessening of security through the growth in zero-hours contracts to about 0.5% as a proportion of the total employment in 2008 to 0.8% in 2012 (ONS, 2013b). These trends illustrate some of the consequences of what Byrne (2005) describes as a qualitative change in the social order in post-industrial society, where business interests dominate politics and, partly as a result, economic insecurity has become a growing feature of more flexible labour markets. This is experienced at an individual level (albeit for those generally towards the bottom of the labour market) and may lead to some of the characteristics of the loss of autonomy and control that Marmot (2004) associated with increased health risks.

More recently Marmot himself contributed to a critique of health risks related to flexible labour markets in the BBC Panorama programme 'Amazon: the truth behind the click'.[42] This provided a powerful insight into the employment practices of a leading retail company using flexible labour and its impact on employee physical and mental health. Marmot stated in the programme that "the characteristics of this type of job, the evidence shows, increase risk of mental illness and physical illness ... There are always going to be menial jobs, but we can make them better or worse. And it seems to me the demands of efficiency at the cost of individual's health and wellbeing – it's got to be balanced." It is worth recalling that Amazon also provides an example of a multinational company seeking to minimise its tax payments in the UK. If we link the potential consequences of its employment practices with its tax arrangements, we see an example of one way in which neoliberal economics can affect health inequalities by both increasing health-related demand and limiting their contribution to health-related costs.

The Big Society appears to be a rather modest response to the structural dynamics relating to the stratification of society described above and in more detail in Chapter Two. For example, 'libertarian paternalism' or 'nudge theory' is a key philosophical strand of the Big Society and promotes the notion that welfare (paternalism) can be promoted while allowing freedom of choice (libertarianism) (Corbett and Walker, 2013). Thaler and Sunstein (2008) contend that here the state can take on the role of 'choice architect' by encouraging schools to arrange food in canteens in such a way as to encourage children to choose healthier food, without banning unhealthy food outright. However, Corbett and Walker (2013) note that nudging people to become 'better' or more successful actors in a market scenario becomes contradictory in the context of market failure, power monopolies, and social and economic inequalities that limit the capability for the poor to participate as equals. Here, they claim that state intervention, regulation and redistribution are necessary. However, Buser highlights how a different approach is being developed: 'bound by a programme of fiscal austerity and a dismantling of the "Big State", mechanisms of civic responsibility, local decision-making and an active third sector are emerging as one means through which public service reform is to be accomplished' (2013: 9). A key concern here for Grimshaw and Rubery (2012) is that not only will austerity measures reverse real spending gains under the previous government but the Big Society vision could also herald a departure from nationally implemented minimum standards.

A further issue is whether the Big Society concept and implementation programmes differentiate sufficiently between varying levels of community capacity in different areas and populations. In practice, not all geographical communities have the same characteristics and strengths. They may be more or less pluralistic in terms of stakeholder interests and more or less cohesive in terms of common purposes, and the latter may vary over time. As Corbett and Walker (2013) argue, the desire for pluralism in the Big Society programme runs counter to the reality of the high concentrations of wealth and power in elite hands and differences in life chances in Britain which there are currently no practical programmes to reverse. If the Big Society conceptually or practically fails to recognise the existence or implications of such variations in capacity and power, there is a risk that the initiatives sponsored under its banner may appear uninviting, irrelevant or excessively onerous to the residents of some communities (see, for example, Dawson, 2013). In turn, this would have consequences for health inequalities in respect of the fit between the incidence of inequalities on the one hand and of community capacity on the other. Similarly, to the extent that community capacity is less extensive or effective than current programmes to address health inequalities, attempts to substitute the latter with the former would risk reducing coverage nationally. In this sense, the complexity and variability of local systems could result in the 'wicked' nature of health inequalities being compounded. Given this background, it is understandable that Evans asserts that:

> The Big Society is a huge natural experiment in public policy with little or no evidence base to support the optimistic claims for the policy made by the Prime Minister or his Secretary of State for Health. There is now an overwhelming body of evidence stretching back from the Black Report in 1980 to the recent Marmot Review that inequalities in wealth are key determinants of inequalities in health. (2011: 11)

As a result, he suggests that by taking £18 billion out of the welfare budget and cutting other public services – which disproportionately benefit for the most disadvantaged in society – government actions will lead to health inequalities between rich and poor widening further.

The significance of policy commitments to localism in tandem with spatial concentrations of health inequalities is considered further elsewhere in this chapter but it is worth underlining the limitations of the Big Society narrative in relation to the uneven spatial distribution of health need and community/neighbourhood capacity to address this. Pearce's argument about the makeup of places reflecting 'broad macrolevel social, economic, and political processes that accumulate over many years' (2013: 2038) is left largely unaddressed by the Coalition's Big Society narrative. In addition, Corbett and Walker assert that the Big Society envisages a role for the state, which 'extends no further than nudging the creation of intermediate institutions for the fulfilment of communal needs, without sufficient attention to existing inequalities, especially in resources such as wealth, time and power' (2013: 460). They cite Hughes Tuohy to highlight how the Big Society appeals to an imagined past consisting of communitarian solidarity and a hierarchical undemocratic order of 'attached unequals', combined with a drastically reduced role for the state. Among others, Buser (2013), Corbett and Walker (2013) and Dawson (2013) are critical of the Big Society for failing to recognise how socioeconomic inequalities in social and economic powers may lead to the more affluent neighbourhoods achieving better outcomes.

Coalition health policy

The Coalition government's major reforms to the NHS were set out in the White Paper *Equity and excellence: Liberating the NHS* in 2010 (DH, 2010b). After a lengthy legislative process, they finally became law in the Health and Social Care Act 2012. The White Paper set out a vision for the NHS, which was described as being rooted in the Coalition's core beliefs of freedom, fairness and responsibility. In doing so it focused on enhancing patient choice, improving clinical outcomes and empowering health professionals. A further aim was to empower patients and the public: 'we will strengthen the collective voice of patients and the public through arrangements led by local authorities, and at national level, through a powerful new consumer champion, HealthWatch England, located in the Care Quality Commission' (DH, 2010b: 3). This emphasis on local government as a vehicle for enhancing the voice of the public on health service matters was not only important in itself but also indicative of an expanded role for local government in the NHS more generally. For the first time since the transfer in 1974 of responsibility for public health and community health services, the White Paper was proposing that local government should have an increased remit for health, including the resumption of responsibility for public health.

Health and Social Care Act 2012

Much of the controversy surrounding the Coalition's health reforms concerned the extent to which they paved the way for the increased commercialisation, if not privatisation, of the publicly funded provision of health services. Concerns among professionals and the general public focused on the role and extent of competition envisaged in the legislation, including its potential for the fragmentation of systems in which improved outcomes were seen to depend on greater collaboration between commissioners and closer integration of supply chains. In particular, the provision that 'any willing provider' should be able to bid for NHS-funded provider contracts was seen by many to open the way for large commercial providers to move into the NHS market (Porter, 2013). By contrast, Timmins argues that such concerns about the extent to which the Health and Social Care Act represented a new direction for the NHS can overlook the trajectory of New Labour policy. He suggests that the legislation can be viewed as 'an extension, a logical outcome even, not just of what Blairite health ministers had been up to but what was intended – or at least implied – way back in 1989 when *Working for Patients* first introduced a quasi-market into the NHS. In the great long sweep of history, it can certainly be viewed in that way' (2012: 126). Even accepting this historical perspective, the implication of Timmins' assessment is still that that the influence of the neoliberal economic model has continued to grow within the NHS and was further reinforced by the Health and Social Care Act 2012. Leaving aside ideological and practical concerns about the commercialisation of health services, these changes have also led to a more fragmented structure of supply of health services. This creates additional organisational complexity within the system, which acts as an added layer of complexity in tackling a set of already wicked problems associated with health inequalities. This analysis is developed further in Chapter Nine.

A further dimension of the White Paper, that of 'liberating the NHS' (DH, 2010b), was its implication for relationships between the NHS and local councils. The document was clear that the achievement of NHS goals depended on that relationship, stating, for example, that it was 'essential for patient outcomes that health and social care services are better integrated at all levels of the system' (DH, 2010b: para 3.11). As a result, the White Paper proposed an expanded role for local government and local democratic accountability in the NHS. Both the White Paper and an accompanying consultation document directly addressed the widely perceived local democratic deficit in the NHS. The latter, entitled *Liberating the NHS: Local democratic legitimacy in health*, envisaged that local authorities would have 'an enhanced role in health' as a result of being allocated 'greater responsibility in four areas:

- leading joint strategic needs assessments (JSNAs) to ensure coherent and co-ordinated commissioning strategies;
- supporting local voice, and the exercise of patient choice;
- promoting joined-up commissioning of local NHS services, social care and health improvement [through health and wellbeing boards (HWBs)]; and
- leading on local health improvement and prevention activity' (DH and DCLG, 2010: para 10).

The same consultation document also saw local authority members bringing greater local democratic legitimacy to health, especially through the HWBs proposed for upper- and single-tier authorities. Although these boards were apparently to be pivotal in 'joining up' commissioning plans, they were also expected to have a substantial role in securing local political and public support for the reconfiguration of hospital services (to the exclusion of scrutiny forums in the initial proposals, although this suggestion was subsequently dropped). In summary, councils would be responsible for taking on health improvement functions from PCTs, coordinating local commissioning and injecting local democratic accountability into a service from which it had been progressively removed between 1974 and 1991.

We now turn to the Health and Social Care Act 2012. Public Health England (PHE) provides a succinct summary of the new arrangements following the introduction of the Act (see Box 6.1).

Box 6.1: New arrangements following the Health and Social Care Act 2012

The implementation of the Health and Social Care Act 2012 has seen the abolition of PCTs and Strategic Health Authorities and the creation of a number of new bodies including Public Health England (PHE), NHS England and Clinical Commissioning Groups (CCGs). At a local level, responsibility for public health has been transferred to local authorities.

The Department of Health (DH) is responsible for strategic leadership of both health and social care systems, but no longer has direct management of most NHS systems. NHS England provides national leadership for improving health

---

care outcomes, directly commissions general practice services, some specialist services and oversees Clinical Commissioning Groups. CCGs now commission planned hospital care, rehabilitative care, urgent and emergency care, most community health services and mental health and learning disability services. Directors of Public Health in Local Authorities are responsible for population health outcomes, supported by PHE, which provides national leadership and expert services to support public health.

Health and Wellbeing Boards act as forums for commissioners across the NHS, social care and public health systems and are responsible for Joint Strategic Needs Assessments and Health and Wellbeing Strategies to inform commissioning. Councillors, especially those with portfolio responsibility for health, have important strategic overview and functions, as well as community engagement and decision-making roles.

Source: PHE (2014a).

Five year forward view

In October 2014 the NHS launched its *Five year forward view*, which advocates a 'radical upgrade in prevention and public health' (NHS, 2014: 9). Furthermore, it makes clear that Wanless' warning 12 years ago that there was a need to take prevention seriously or the country would be faced with a sharply rising burden of avoidable illness has not been heeded. This is significant, given our earlier argument about the dominant logic model of the NHS being too narrowly focused on health (medical) care for all, rather than on health for all. Indeed, it is reassuring that the *Five year forward view* recognises that 'if the nation fails to get serious about prevention then ... health inequalities will widen, and our ability to fund beneficial new treatments will be crowded out by the need to spend billions of pounds on wholly avoidable illness' (NHS, 2014: 7). This, in turn, would continue to divert the focus of the NHS away from tackling the social and economic determinants of health inequalities.

Drivers for change in public health

When the Royal Society for Public Health (RSPH) reviewed the new landscape for public health following the passage of the 2012 Act it identified three key drivers for change in public health (RSPH, 2014: 8):

- the Marmot Review, which highlights the disparity in life expectancy between individuals and communities;
- *Healthy lives, healthy people*, (DH, 2012) which details the transfer of primary public health responsibilities to local authorities;
- the localism agenda, which gives councils more freedom to work together with others in new ways to drive down costs. It seeks to give them increased confidence to do innovative things to meet local needs.

We explore each of these in more detail in the following subsections.

Marmot Review and the Coalition government

In Chapter One we drew attention to the Marmot Review (2010) and how this highlighted the vast social gradients in health that have become entrenched in the UK, so that those in the poorest areas will die on average seven years younger than those in the richest, and spend 17 more years living with a disability. We then moved on to summarise the key behavioural risk factors for ill health identified by the Review and the areas identified as being particularly powerful in shaping health and health inequalities – the 'causes of the causes' or 'social determinants of health'. Chapter four of the Review followed up this analysis by setting out detailed policy and priority objectives that are grouped under six areas and are summarised in Table 6.1 overleaf. It is worth recalling the changing political context for the Review: it was commissioned by the Labour government in 2008 but within three months of being published a Conservative/Liberal Democrat Coalition government was in place. Bambra et al (2011) note that an awareness of a changing political context may have shaped the way the Review was drafted and led to some rather vague and diluted recommendations, in order to remain acceptable to different ideological perspectives and avoid the marginalisation that befell the Black Report.

The Marmot Review states that 'delivering these policy objectives will require action by central and local government, the NHS, the third and private sectors and community groups. National policies will not work without effective local delivery systems focused on health equity in all policies' (2010: 15). Allen (2013) argues that there has been widespread uptake and endorsement of the Marmot Review's approach and recommendations, with the 2011 public health White Paper (HM Government, 2010b) and subsequent Public Health Outcomes Framework being heavily influenced by this. Locally, over 75% of local authorities are working to embed the Marmot principles

Table 6.1: Marmot Review – policy and priority objectives

Policy objective	Priority objectives
Give every child the best start in life	Reduce inequalities in the early development of physical and emotional health, and cognitive, linguistic, and social skills. Ensure high quality maternity services, parenting programmes, childcare and early years education to meet needs across the social gradient. Build the resilience and well-being of young children across the social gradient.
Enable all children, young people and adults to maximise their capabilities and have greater control over their lives	Reduce the social gradient in skills and qualifications. Ensure that schools, families and communities work in partnership to reduce the gradient in health, well-being and resilience of children and young people. Improve the access and use of quality lifelong learning across the social gradient.
Create fair employment and good work for all	Improve access to good jobs and reduce long-term unemployment across the social gradient. Make it easier for people who are disadvantaged in the labour market to obtain and keep work. Improve quality of jobs across the social gradient.
Ensure healthy living standard for all	Establish a minimum income for healthy living for people of all ages. Reduce the social gradient in the standard of living through progressive taxation and other fiscal policies. Reduce the cliff edges faced by people moving between benefits and work.
Create and develop healthy and sustainable communities	Develop common policies to reduce the scale and impact of climate change and health inequalities. Improve community capital and reduce social isolation across the social gradient.
Strengthen the role and impact of ill health prevention	Prioritise prevention and early detection of those conditions most strongly related to health inequalities. Increase availability of long-term and sustainable funding in ill health prevention across the social gradient.

Source: Marmot Review (2010)..

in their approaches to improve health and reduce inequalities (Allen, 2013). Humphries and Galea's (2013) survey of English local authorities found that the six policy objectives were the most frequently mentioned priorities agreed by HWBs. As a result, the Marmot Review appears to have had a real impact across local health and care systems. However, it is at the national level (and despite the government accepting most of its recommendations) that Gregory et al (2012) highlight an important exception: the prescription to narrow income inequalities. Indeed, the Marmot Review was explicit in making a strong connection between 'social inequalities in health [and] inequalities in the conditions of daily life and the fundamental drivers that give rise to them: inequities in power, money and resources' (2010: 16). Accordingly, it stated that:

> These social and economic inequalities underpin the determinants of health: the range of interacting factors that shape health and well-being. These include: material circumstances, the social environment, psychological factors, behaviours, and biological factors. In turn, these factors are influenced by social position, itself shaped by education, occupation, income, gender, ethnicity and race. All these influences are shaped by the socio-political and cultural and social context in which they sit. (2010: 16)

The quotation from the Marmot Review outlines a position that would sit comfortably within the European conception of 'equality of condition', which was discussed in Chapter Two (in the section on inequality). In other words, there needs to be an explicit challenge to significant divisions of power, wealth and security, as these are essentially the 'drivers' of health inequalities. However, Finlayson (2010) contends that at the core of Coalition policy there is an effort to refute claims that economic processes (in particular, economic inequalities) have social effects. According to David Cameron, the crisis facing Britain is one of individuals failing to take responsibility for themselves, each other or their society (caused by the social democratic state limiting the notion of self-reliance), rather than the effects of neoliberal competitiveness and inequality (Finlayson, 2010). This strong possessive individualist strand to Cameron's philosophy, which has important implications for how health inequalities are framed under the Coalition government – that is, that health inequalities are a concern for government but, somewhat contradictorily, from a position in which individual rights have predominance over collective rights and inequality is deemed a natural function of society. This apparent contradiction can be illustrated through the 'health premium', which was introduced under the DH's (2012) *Healthy lives, healthy people: Improving outcomes and supporting transparency*, and will be awarded to areas linked to rates of improvement for health and risk indicators in an outcomes framework linked to healthy life expectancy. This is part of the government's strategy to 'improve the health of the poorest the fastest'. However, Barr et al (2012) highlight the importance of historical socioeconomic conditions for health improvement and the likely slower rates of economic growth and improvements in life expectancy in socioeconomically deprived areas. Consequently, the health premium may be regressive, as the challenge to improve health is likely to be greater in deprived areas and, therefore, tends to be associated with slower rates of health improvement, which could lead to resources moving away from these areas (Barr et al, 2012). So, while the Coalition government has embraced much of the Marmot Review's findings and, in so doing, adopted an approach towards health inequalities that apparently recognises the interactions between individual and social levels of explanation, it also intensifies a trend for what Glasby (2012) describes as official responses falling short of the initial diagnosis of health inequalities (as with the Black Report).

Transfer of public health responsibilities to local government

In *Healthy lives, healthy people* the intention to place local government and local communities 'at the heart of improving health and wellbeing for their populations and tackling inequalities' is made explicit (HM Government, 2010b: 4). The Health and Social Care Act 2012 gave local authorities a core role in public health, with dedicated funding ($£2.5$ billion in 2013/14) and support from a new executive agency, PHE, and a new Public Health Outcomes Framework (Buck and Gregory, 2013). The Framework sets out what the Coalition government wants to achieve in a new and reformed public health system (DH, 2012). It focuses on two high-level outcomes: increasing healthy life expectancy and reducing differences between communities in health outcomes.

Under the Health and Social Care Act 2012, local authorities have the lead role in tackling avoidable health inequalities in health outcomes (Gregory et al, 2012), which relates to the shift in responsibility for public health services. The RSPH, citing the DH, describes local authority public health commissioning responsibilities as including:

> tobacco control; alcohol and drug misuse services; public health services for children (5–19 years); national child measurement programme; obesity programme; nutrition initiatives; physical activity; NHS health check assessments; public mental health; dental public health; accident injury prevention; population level interventions to reduce birth defects; behavioural programmes to reduce cancer and long term conditions; workplace health; immunisation and screening; sexual health services; initiatives to reduce mortality from seasonal issues (cold/heat deaths); health

protection including protection from environmental risks; community safety; and tackling social exclusion. (2014: 15)

While these responsibilities do not explicitly refer to health inequalities there is considerable overlap with the main behavioural risk factors for ill health outlined in Chapter One (in the section on potential causes). Consequently, when added to local government's role in education, social care and community and neighbourhood development, responsibility for two of the three areas the NAO (2010) identifies as being causes of health inequalities (wider determinants and the lives people lead) are key features of local government's duties. Indeed, Buck and Gregory's review of the literature sets out nine areas in which there is strong evidence that local authorities can improve public health and reduce inequalities. These are:

- the best start in life;
- healthy schools and pupils;
- helping people find good jobs and stay in work;
- active and safe travel;
- warmer and safer homes;
- access to green and open spaces and the role of leisure services;
- strong communities, wellbeing and resilience;
- public protection and regulatory services (including takeaway/fast food, air pollution, and fire safety); and
- health and spatial planning (2013: 1).

As this list of functions and responsibilities illustrates, the new landscape for public health is one which has the potential to integrate public health with other core responsibilities related to the social determinants of health within a single local organisation. The RSPH notes that 'traditionally, commissioning has been focused on service targets and that has been interpreted as a focus on distinct topics – e.g. smoking, weight loss, exercise ... this has tended to squeeze out commissioning for those aspects of strategic social and community development that have longer term, positive and sustainable impacts on health states' (2014: 20). It continues by pointing out that local authorities are in a position to build health-enabling communities, where healthy behaviours are the norm and are firmly rooted in improving the social context of their populations through influencing local social customs and norms and the physical environment. Turner et al (2013: 7) also identify some optimism here, as local authorities have more of a track record of focusing on equality in housing and education provision. However, Craig (2013) argues that the changing role for local government will be challenging, as health has spread across two separate sectors that have historically struggled to integrate. Indeed, Wistow (2012) contends that a fundamental weakness of the current arrangements is that they were built around the skills of the providers rather than the needs of users, and for the purpose of separation rather than integration.

Despite these continuing concerns about integration, local authorities have shifted from junior partners in public health to now hosting public health departments, and they operate HWBs, which oversee the development of JSNAs and joint health and wellbeing strategies. The Health and Social Care Act 2012 sets out the functions of HWBs as a statutory committee of the local authority and specifies their core memberships but permits flexibility in how they are set up and operated (Humphries and Galea, 2013). In *Equity and excellence* it was stated that HWBs would 'allow local authorities to take a strategic approach and promote integration across health and adult social care, children's services, including safeguarding, and the wider local authority agenda' (DH, 2010b: 34). As a result, HWBs are the local forums where systems leaders from local government, the NHS and other interests could come together to improve health and wellbeing outcomes and reduce health inequalities. In practice, however, HWBs have no powers to approve – or otherwise – local commissioning plans, and despite attempts to enhance their powers they remain poorly equipped to operate in a systems leadership or management role (Wistow, 2011; 2012, House of Commons Health Committee, 2012).

The localism agenda

The section on the Big Society above outlined a key philosophical strand of the Coalition government's policy that has particular relevance for localism. Here, we return to this theme and focus on localism more generally and how this might relate to health inequalities. The Localism Bill 2010 devolves 'power, money and knowledge to those best placed to find the best solutions to local needs: elected local representatives, frontline public service professionals, social enterprises, charities, co-ops, community groups, neighbourhoods and individuals' (HM Government, 2010a: 2). Similarly, in *Healthy lives, healthy people* it is stated that 'localism will be at the heart of this [public health] system, with responsibilities, freedoms and funding devolved wherever possible' (HM Government, 2010b: 8). Castelli et al (2013) argue that the nature of these changes means that we should look beyond usual geographic levels of regional, local authority or health district area to smaller geographical areas that may be more representative of local communities or neighbourhoods. Buck and Gregory agree, and note that 'giving communities more power over neighbourhood-level plans, which councils are obliged to support ... provides an excellent opportunity for neighbourhood-level planning for health and use of community assets' (2013: 3).

Local authorities now have a statutory responsibility for improving the health of their people and the NHS's (2014) *Five year forward view* states that they should be granted enhanced powers to allow local democratic decisions on public health policy affecting physical and mental health. PHE (2014b) published a sister document, *From evidence into action: Opportunities to protect and improve the nation's health*, which sets out seven key priorities to change individuals' lifestyles. These are tackling obesity, reducing smoking, reducing harmful drinking, ensuring every child has the best start in life, reducing dementia risk, tackling antimicrobial resistance and reducing tuberculosis. It acknowledges that our health is shaped by where and how we live but that individuals have the power to change the way they live, and that to do so the ideas underpinning the key priorities must take root locally, in people's neighbourhoods and communities.

Craig draws attention to the potential to be derived from more closely connecting HWBs to their communities: 'public services today do a great deal to care for people in distress or in trouble: they could do a great deal more to help them improve their lives and help them avoid times of distress and trouble. Public services that build and utilise assets within people, connect people and foster flourishing communities are the kind that build better societies' (2013: 4). However, at this point, it remains unclear how far HWBs will be able to develop the close connections with their communities necessary to realise this potential. The success or otherwise of initiatives like that sponsored by 'Think local act personal' to promote the community capacity-building role of HWBs should begin to provide indicators of how much progress can be made in practice.

It is helpful here to unpack some of the additional challenges that face socioeconomically deprived areas. Pearce (2012) identifies four individualised and institutionalised pathways that might compromise population health and health inequalities through spatial stigma.

- Feeling 'looked down on' because of external perceptions of stigmatised communities may lead to limited opportunities for education, training, employment and interpersonal relationships.

- Place-based stigma can act as a 'badge of dishonour' that may spoil, mediate and manipulate individual identities and social relations, which in turn can affect physical and mental health–related behaviours.
- Disinvestment of public and private resources in the local community and infrastructure can undermine progressive social policy that provides opportunities for healthy living.
- Residents may withdraw from the public realm, affecting local social networks and bonds, which may be detrimental to physical and mental health.

Pearce's argument about the 'blemish of place' draws attention to a key issue that is arguably largely neglected through the Coalition government's policy on health inequalities and localism: that socioeconomic context matters, both in terms of the scale of the challenge and the capacity to address that challenge. Consequently, Castelli et al's (2013) summary of the Coalition's policy shift to, first, increasingly emphasising the local dimension in many areas of public policy making (including health); and second, giving local authorities new responsibilities to reflect their role in influencing the health and wellbeing of their populations should be considered alongside the resources necessary to fulfil such responsibilities. In this respect, the programme of austerity discussed above provides a troubling backdrop, which has led authors such as Lowndes and Pratchett to describe the Coalition's approach to localism as 'sink or swim', with the impact of the cuts likely to undermine the prospects of 'all but the most affluent areas' (2012: 37–8).

Implications for health inequalities

We now turn to potential implications and concerns about health inequalities under the Coalition government's health policy. Given that, at the time of writing, statistics for health inequalities for the last year of the New Labour government are still unavailable, the analysis here cannot be definitive in respect of the inherited baseline. Nevertheless, based on what we know about the causes of health inequalities (see, for example, Marmot, 2010; NAO, 2010), we can draw on recent literature to offer a general and qualified critique of the direction of travel under the Coalition government and potential implications for health inequalities. Turner et al's (2013: 7) research provides a useful summary of three key concerns identified by health and social care commissioners regarding the Coalition government's commitment to health inequalities. These are weakened directives from central government, clinical commissioners' lack of engagement with population perspectives and reduced public health input into health service commissioning. We use these themes to structure this section and expand on Turner et al's analysis.

Weakened directives from central government

The role of the DH, its ministers and central government agencies more generally in relation to health inequalities has to be viewed in the context of the current administration's criticisms of detailed performance management from the centre. In the NHS, it specifically wished to reduce what it saw as the dysfunctional impact of targets and the over-detailed interventions of ministers in the day-to-day operation of the service. In *Equity and excellence* it was asserted that 'the NHS will be held to account against clinically credible and evidence-based outcome measures, not process targets. We will remove targets with no clinical justification' (DH, 2010b: 4). The Health and Social Care Act 2012 made some controversial changes to the responsibilities of the Secretary of State (see below) and also created the national NHS Commissioning Board (now known as NHS England) as an agency at arm's length from the DH and the Secretary of State. The Board exercises responsibility for the NHS by setting outcomes against which its performance is assessed and a mandate, laid before parliament annually, setting out expectations of progress across a number of domains of activity. One implication of this division of responsibilities is that a less directive and engaged role for the centre, and especially the DH, was built into the 2012 Act. Changes in central/local relations in respect of health inequalities thus need to be assessed in the light of this wider governance agenda, as well as for their possible indications of changes in policies, priorities and delivery systems specifically directed at health inequalities. How far the implications of the new governance regime for reducing inequalities were considered and understood is another matter. However, it is interesting to note that the Public Health Minister was recorded in June 2013 as saying: "I don't know how much any of you realise that with the Lansley Act we pretty much gave away control of the NHS, which means that [for] the thing that most people talk about in terms of health [the NHS] ... we have some important strategic mechanisms but we don't really have day-to-day control" (Helm, 2014).

We begin this section by drawing on the work of Gregory et al, who identify three areas of action that the DH is supporting:

- funding the Marmot Review team to continue collecting evidence and to offer expert advice (especially to local authorities) on how action on the wider determinants of health can reduce health inequalities;
- instituting a cross-government health inequalities programme review board; and
- continuing to support the previous government's inclusion health policy, seeking to drive improvements in health outcomes for social excluded groups (2012: 46–7).

Despite these developments there is a consistent theme in the literature highlighting concern about weakened directives from central government in relation to health inequalities. Bovaird et al highlight that 'while the Coalition government's documents consistently emphasise continued commitment to outcome-based working, it has a much more fragmented approach to setting and measuring outcomes in local public services, especially since the abolition of the national indicator set' (2014: 553). Staite and Miller (2011) argue that this is particularly confusing in relation to health and wellbeing. For example, the government has stopped performance managing localities on the life expectancy and infant mortality targets, but continues to monitor these. However, the 18–week target for hospital treatment remains in force and has been embedded in the NHS constitution, as do targets for cancer care, while the DH still pays close attention to waiting times as a key performance measure (Gregory et al, 2012), and both the Prime Minister and Health Secretary are known to have been personally involved in the weekly monitoring of accident and emergency attendances and emergency admissions to hospital. Notwithstanding the context of the new framework for central/local relations initiated by the 2012 Act, therefore, these examples consistently appear to point to a greater relaxation in relation to public health and health inequalities than to aspects of acute medicine.

Through the Health and Social Care Act 2012, para 13G, the NHS Commissioning Board is required to 'reduce inequalities between patients with respect to their ability to access health services, and reduce inequalities between patients with respect to the outcomes achieved for them by the provision of health services'. The subsequent *The mandate: A mandate from the government to the NHS Commissioning Board: April 2013 to March 2015* refers to the NHS Commissioning Board's duties to reduce unjustifiable inequalities in access to services, the quality of care received and the outcomes from that care (DH, 2013). Gregory et al (2012: 46) argue that while the Board will be held to account for progress in reducing health inequalities, the limited detail about how this will be measured and assessed means that the objective lacks robustness. Pollock et al contend that 'the [Health and Social Care] Bill severs the duty of the Secretary of State for Health to secure comprehensive health care throughout England and introduces competitive markets and structures consistent with greater inequality of provision, mixed funding, and widespread provision by private health corporations' (2012: 1). They point out that considerable discretionary powers will be granted to commissioners and providers of care, where once there was a statutory duty to provide comprehensive health care. As a result, it is unclear whether the new legal duties relating to health inequalities will be able to counter the increased variation that the move to a more local NHS (as CCGs take decisions about what to fund at a local level) is likely to lead. However, Gregory et al (2012) assert that the new NHS Commissioning Board is in strong position, as the new monopoly purchaser of primary care, to monitor these duties rigorously and ensure that interventions are targeted towards a fast reduction in health inequalities (as set out in the NAO, 2010 report).

The NAO identifies that 'the three interventions which the Department has shown can improve life expectancy, by preventing or reducing the risk of ill health, and which were to be implemented from 2007 are:

- increase the prescribing of drugs to control blood pressure by 40 per cent;
- increase the prescribing of drugs to reduce cholesterol by 40 per cent; and
- double the capacity of smoking cessation services' (2010: 10).

These three interventions reflect areas in which the DH estimates that around 15–20% of inequalities in mortality rates can be directly influenced by health interventions. This is not an insignificant space for action, but it does also reflect the rather narrow focus of personal medical services in framing health inequality interventions.

A further issue relates to the lack of clarity about roles of organisations in the reformed health and social care system. Indeed, confusion about roles in the new system was identified in Humphries and Galea's (2013) research as the biggest factor impeding progress (alongside the financial climate). PHE will support local authorities in carrying out public health responsibilities, but will not performance manage or intervene to the extent that the NHS Commissioning Board is likely to with the NHS. Gregory et al conclude by arguing that a matching health inequalities duty should have been placed on local authorities to 'ensure that both leading players on health and wellbeing boards have matching and consistent duties on inequality reduction' (2012: 47). Jessica Allen (former project director for Marmot Review and current deputy director of the Institute of Health Equity[43]) notes that the effects of reorganisation have meant that health inequalities seem to have slipped, or may be slipping, off many agendas. Allen (2013) claims that the NHS Commissioning Board, PHE and the DH all need to lead action and focus on health inequalities but, perhaps due to the demands of reorganisation, it is unclear where the necessary leadership and focus will come from.

Furthermore, the continuing existence of three separate but interrelated outcomes frameworks for social care, public health and the NHS, rather than a single unified framework, is highlighted by Wistow as a signal of integration remaining on the margins of NHS and local government because their mainstream business is defined in terms of delivering individual services or functions. He points out that 'unfortunately, no one below the Secretary of State and his Cabinet colleagues has the duty or means to deliver a differently balanced care system' (2012: 111).

Clinical commissioners' lack of engagement with population perspectives

In *Equity and excellence* (DH, 2010b) it was argued that the closer involvement of GPs in the commissioning of care would ensure effective dialogue between primary and secondary care, move decision making closer to the patient and increase efficiency (Checkland et al, 2013). However, there are also concerns about this change to commissioning arrangements owing to fears that CCGs will not engage sufficiently with population perspectives. For example, the RSPH states that health improvement for disadvantaged groups needs to raise those social aspects of life that promote and enhance health status and wellbeing, and that this 'requires a particular form of approach and understanding of how to promote health as opposed to treating or preventing disease or illness' (2014: 11).

Checkland et al cite Miller et al (2012) to assert that 'previous GP commissioners have tended to focus on areas of activity based on their direct experiences as clinicians ... there is limited evidence of engagement with a public health approach' (2013: 612). Turner et al's (2013) research supports this argument, as their analysis indicated it was likely that there would be piecemeal attention to health inequalities at best, with GPs generally drawing on experiences of the consultancy room, which would undermine attention on under-served groups. In addition, the NAO (2010) highlighted that a lot of people who are expected to have key health conditions are not recorded on GP registers. The Health Inequalities National Support Team (HINST) describes this problem as 'the missing thousands' (see Chapter Seven, section on practical illustrations), where the level of expressed demand recorded on GPs registers does not correspond to the actual level of need.

Checkland et al (2013) note that CCGs have ambitions to move beyond commissioning, focused on the immediate needs of registered patients, but there is little concrete evidence of new approaches as yet. Indeed, Miller et al (2012) highlight that most change in primary care commissioning since the introduction of a quasi-market in the NHS has been associated with things closely related to, or under the direct control of, primary care, such as prescribing and improving services related to primary care. As a result, Turner et al (2013) conclude that while it is likely that CCGs will take a much more person-centred approach, there are concerns about their understanding of the importance of taking a population perspective on inequalities and about CCGs overlooking the need for effective community engagement. Taken together, there are a range of challenges for CCGs that represent a sharp learning curve for groups that have, by their nature, a medical view of health. Consequently, it may reasonably be expected that it will, at best, take time for CCGs to adjust to commissioning for population, as opposed to patient, health.

A further issue identified by Dorling (2013a) is that under the Health and Social Care Act 2012 the duty to provide comprehensive care was transferred from the Secretary of State to CCGs; this is likely to lead to a further concentration of spatial inequalities in health care as more affluent areas tend to have more to spend. Turner et al (2013: 11) note that the proposal to link funding formulas solely to the age of the population, rather than including area deprivation as well, makes it increasingly important not only to understand the scale of inequalities but to fight for resources to address them. However, at the time of writing NHS England is reviewing the NHS allocations process, having rejected proposed changes to the current allocations formula as being inconsistent with its duty to reduce health inequalities. There are also concerns about GPs being the most effective advocates for prioritising health inequalities. For example, Dorling points out that 'when health inequalities are high and there are large variations between areas, doctors appear not to want to live in areas with high health needs'

(2013a: 12). Nevertheless, Gregory et al (2012: 43) contend that the role of the NHS has been strengthened in this respect through the legal role to reduce inequalities in access to care and the outcomes from that care, but with less responsibility for tackling overall inequalities in health. Consequently, this might be interpreted as a continuation of the narrowly focused logic model of the NHS – one which we described in Chapter Five as a category error in terms of focusing on improvements in access to health rather than improvements in health itself.

Reduced public health input into health service commissioning

Turner et al (2013) highlight concerns about the extent to which the new commissioners will be able to work in partnership, engage and exert the necessary influence over the system. There is some optimism reported in their findings that primary care will improve as shared backgrounds on CCGs may lead to cooperation in areas in which PCTs struggled in the past. But this did not stretch to respondents'[44] confidence about working with hospitals, where many thought they would be out of their depth. The move of public health to local authorities was seen, by some respondents, as potentially leading to greater integration of knowledge and data, and stronger JSNAs and understanding of health needs. Despite these positive views, the more general feeling was that restructuring presented significant risks to partnership working – time to build trust and limited experience of GPs working in partnership were identified as key factors here (especially GPs' lack of understanding about how local authorities work) (Turner et al, 2013).

Coleman et al (2014) show that the Health and Social Care Act states that CCGs and the NHS Commissioning Board must give regard to HWBs when carrying out their functions, but that this does not extend to any formal authority for HWBs to veto or change CCG plans. Indeed, as has been argued above, HWBs appear to be poorly equipped to adopt a systems leader role. Turner et al (2013) also identify a 'worrying theme' of historically poor relationships between GPs, public health colleagues, local authorities and the third sector that may limit the impact of clinical commissioning beyond primary care and undermine the scope for HWBs to get deep cross-sectoral commitment to inequalities work. However, Turner et al also recognise the variability of these relationships across areas, with some being much better than those described above. They identify some hopes among their respondents that HWB services will be more accountable to local communities and that through strengthened JSNAs more coordinated work to address social and economic determinants will result from public health's move to local authorities.

A further concern identified by Gregory et al, (2012) relates to the 2013/14 NHS resource allocations, which will be separated from the allocations for public health: the King's Fund anticipates this will be a rough 95% and 5% split between the two, respectively. Consequently, Gregory et al argue that this may lead to a reduction in inequalities in access to care but an overall increase in health outcome inequalities. The House of Commons Health Committee (2014) expressed concern that following reorganisation there is reduced capacity in the public health workforce due to unfulfilled posts. This may affect the role of public health in commissioning services. The Committee also expressed some apprehension that PHE had been slow to establish a prioritised programme of work. In addition, it was concerned that Duncan Selbie, PHE's Chief Executive, regarded it as 'too controversial' to address the question of health inequalities when giving evidence to the Committee. The Committee concluded that there is insufficient separation between PHE and the DH, and that the voice of PHE had not been heard clearly enough, as yet. Again, we return to the significance of the personal medicine paradigm and the dominance of this logic model within health service commissioning. If the national public health agency is unable to distance itself from the DH, there is a danger that the historic category error in the development of the NHS will be repeated across the new arrangements, and that the 'causes of the causes' of health inequalities and the socially and economically structured patterns of these determinants of health will continue to be neglected, relative to the personal medicine paradigm.

Conclusion

Much of the discussion in this chapter has necessarily been framed by the financial crisis, the subsequent austerity programme and a shift towards a more libertarian approach to governance. Indeed, Lupton et al concluded that the Coalition's:

> agenda for government comprises not only reduced public spending but a restructuring of the welfare state incorporating a reduction in the size and functions of government at all levels, less central policy direction, a shift to private and/or voluntary provision of public goods, and less generous welfare benefits, including greater conditionality. (2013: 8)

Thus, Clarke and Newman (2012) assert that political rationalisations of the Coalition programme have moved uncomfortably between the claim of economic necessity and a more moral and social vocabulary of responsibility and interdependence.

The backdrop to local authorities and communities being given much greater freedom to organise and prioritise services is one in which (already high) levels of inequality are likely to increase. Pearce (2013) contends that the reduction in spending power among local authorities is likely to lead to an increasingly divergent quality in services, and that this may undermine the local infrastructures that influence health through health promotion, community networks and a multitude of other pathways. Pearce concludes that 'as more powerful and skilled interest groups work to shield themselves from the material implications of fiscal tightening, residents of low-income communities are therefore likely to be disproportionately affected by the reduced investment in neighbourhood infrastructure' (2013: 2039). Similarly, Dawson (2013) notes that the Big Society does not address inequalities, as individuals are likely to seek the best for their own neighbourhoods without placing these within a wider social concern, leading to a 'postcode lottery', in which the more affluent neighbourhoods are more likely to be effective in fulfilling their 'sectional desires'.

Taking all these observations together in the light of the analysis of policy earlier in this chapter, it seems necessary to recognise a potentially fundamental contradiction in policies to reduce health inequalities and a fiscal regime built on macroeconomic policies which reinforce economic inequalities, together with resource allocation policies for public expenditure that are affecting areas of high socioeconomic inequality most unfavourably. In addition, the attempt to square the circle of fiscal austerity and growing health needs through community capacity building and the Big Society are likely to be most challenging in precisely those areas where health inequalities are more serious. The immediate prospects for addressing health inequalities effectively seem, therefore, more limited than under the previous administration which, itself, in a much more favourable policy environment, was unable to achieve a closing of the gap between geographical areas.

Part Three
Case studies

SEVEN

Evidence for public health practice: Health Inequalities National Support Team

Chris Bentley and Peter Counsell

Introduction

This chapter is a case study that summarises the learning from a team that worked with local partnerships in the most deprived areas of England to reduce health inequalities – the Health Inequalities National Support Team (HINST). The team used two underpinning models that are congruent with the underlying thesis of this book – that work to address health inequalities and the complex dynamic relationships that support the status quo (Figures 7.3 and 7.4, pp 160, 163). The chapter provides practical examples of approaches to reduce health inequalities and effective practice at a local level. Appendix A links to the practical techniques developed by the Team. Although the structure of statutory agencies charged with addressing health inequalities has changed, the principles remain relevant, and the chapter provides a case study of the practical issues encountered when the underlying theses of this book are applied to practice.

From 2007 until it was closed down by the Coalition government in 2011, HINST operated on the premise that it is possible to narrow gaps in health outcomes by targeting local policy and action, which is one of the principle themes explored in this book, as outlined in the first chapter. Its aim was to promote effective practice in this area of public health, as a resource in public health practice for academics, researchers and public health practitioners. Much of what follows can be viewed in terms of issues around the boundaries, dynamics, self-organisation and co-evolution of systems involved in addressing health inequalities. As such, the chapter makes implicit connections to the complexity-based framing of this book, and these connections are reflected upon more explicitly in the concluding chapter.

The chapter begins by providing a brief introduction to the context and evolution of HINST, which includes an overview of the Team's programme, a summary of its evolution and some reflections on the health inequality outcomes. The next section provides a more detailed account of the principles that underpinned the HINST approach. The following section provides a series of practical illustrations of effective practice identified by HINST. The changing environment under the Coalition government is then considered, with a focus on requirements for delivering population-level change through the new policy structure. The chapter concludes with some reflections on how the HINST model can be capitalised on.

Context and evolution of HINST

The national support teams programme

From 2006, the Department of Health (DH) established ten thematic national support teams to support local areas in tackling complex public health issues using the best available evidence. They operated within a shared framework, adopting similar processes based on a common model of change.

The national support team process involved a pre-visit desk review of selected documentation and data-based intelligence, followed by interviews with key informants, often in combination with a series of workshops or focus groups. Collation and analysis of findings was immediate, and the findings – including strengths and recommendations – were fed back straight away to the key local players at each site. Recommendations were accompanied by offers of support, either at the time of reporting or as through a package of follow-up activity to address agreed priorities.

The national support teams were appointed as change agents. Iles and Sutherland's National Health Service (NHS) manual on organisational change underpinning this approach encouraged the teams to challenge the 'implicit assumptions that dictate the direction of seemingly disparate and unrelated decisions, (that) shape the change process by emergent rather than "planned" change' (2001: 14).

The evolution of HINST

HINST was founded in 2007 with the explicit purpose of helping the local teams working in the most deprived fifth of local authority areas to reduce the gap in health inequalities. It worked, therefore, with the 70 Spearhead areas. These were selected on the basis that they fell into the lowest quintile of all English local authorities in at least three of the following five criteria:

- male life expectancy at birth;
- female life expectancy at birth;
- cancer mortality rate in under–75s;
- cardiovascular disease (CVD) mortality rate in under–75s;
- Index of Multiple Deprivation 2004 (Local Authority Summary), average score.

The 70 Spearhead areas were in the North, the Midlands and London (see Figure 7.1).

Figure 7.1: Map of Spearhead areas

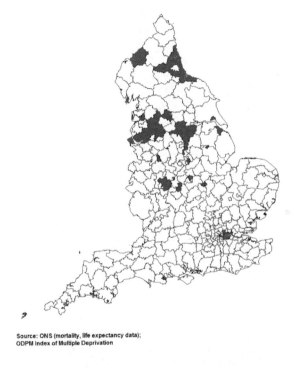

Source: ONS (mortality, life expectancy data);
ODPM Index of Multiple Deprivation

HINST worked to an explicit public service agreement (PSA) target, which was refined over time to include a mixture of improvements in absolute terms (such as mortality rates), and relative terms (such as the gap in inequalities between authority areas). As the PSA target deadline of 2010 came closer there was a discernible change of focus in the recommendations made through this target, emphasising those things that would make a difference to the target population in the time that remained.

- Interventions were recommended that had to be applied systematically and on an 'industrial' scale to have sufficient impact on life expectancy at a population level.
- The potential impact of interventions on the number of lives to be saved was calculated, enabling choices about local priorities and the scale of change against investment to be planned.
- There was an intensified focus on health service changes that could be made which would add years of life to those who were otherwise facing an early death.

Recommendations made by HINST to the Spearheads it visited included a balance of actions ranging from those that would have an immediate impact (within the timeframe of the PSA target) through to those which would have a more sustained impact over time, as Figure 7.2 shows.

The lessons that had been learned about delivering short-term targets

Figure 7.2: Different gestation times for interventions[45]

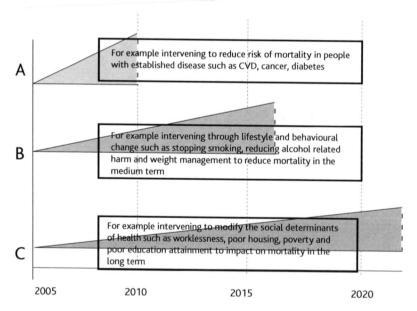

For example intervening to reduce risk of mortality in people with established disease such as CVD, cancer, diabetes

For example intervening through lifestyle and behavioural change such as stopping smoking, reducing alcohol related harm and weight management to reduce mortality in the medium term

For example intervening to modify the social determinants of health such as worklessness, poor housing, poverty and poor education attainment to impact on mortality in the long term

2005   2010   2015   2020

were necessary to inform the development of strategies to address medium- and long-term goals. These include the need to focus on system, scale and sustainability, and what mechanisms might deliver given interventions to achieve these necessary attributes for population level change.

The outcome

Following the change in government in 2010 the PSA target was dropped in favour of local targets before the end of its timeframe, and national monitoring ceased. However, the Public Health leadership in North West Region maintained their component of the national target as an interim measure, while local targets were developed, and analysis has continued there. This shows that the Spearhead life expectancy target would not have been reached within the timeframe planned, but there were some successes.

The best analysis so far is given by Tom Hennell, Senior Public Health Analyst, Department of Health North West[46] in a presentation that concludes:

The good news

- The national Spearhead target for male life expectancy appears to have been met in 2009–2011.
- Although the national Spearhead target for female life expectancy appears to have been missed in 2009–2011, there are signs of narrowing gaps since 2006–2008.
- Whatever interventions Spearhead areas have been applying to reduce inequalities in public health over the last four years, they should keep them up, because they're working.
- The three cause-specific objective targets for 2010 were achieved in Spearheads in areas in 2009.

The bad news

- Progress is locally variable; with the most successful narrowing of gaps in London and the North East.
- Improvement in the female cancer mortality gap is badly lagging that for the male cancer mortality gap.

Principles that underpin the HINST approach

Principles for intervention

HINST evolved through its interaction with local teams – drawing on and disseminating a growing body of effective practice to underpin its recommendations. The team emphasised that interventions within a given population by a given date would require systematic programmes of action that are known to be effective and reaching as many of the target audience of people as possible who could benefit.

Programme characteristics included being:

- evidence-based – concentrating on interventions where research findings and professional consensus are strongest;
- outcomes-oriented – with measurements locally relevant and locally owned;
- systematically applied – not depending on exceptional circumstances and exceptional champions;scaled up appropriately – 'industrial-scale' processes require different thinking from small-scale projects or pilots ('bench experiments');
- appropriately resourced – refocusing on core budgets and services rather than short bursts of project funding;
- persistent – continuing for the long haul, capitalising on, but not dependent on fads, fashion and changing policy priorities.

Interventions can be delivered through three different approaches to drive change (focused on the population, individual and community levels) as illustrated by Figure 7.3.

Figure 7.3: Three approaches to population-level change

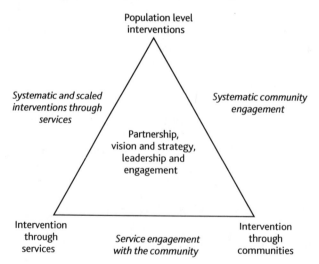

Three approaches to population-level change

Population approaches

Direct population-level interventions include developing healthy public policy, legislation, regulation, taxation and public funding strategies. These elements should support making 'healthy choices easy choices' for individuals and communities.

The impacts of such population-level interventions, however, will not automatically 'trickle down' to everyone, often missing those who are socially excluded for various reasons. Strategies for targeted communication and education, service support and even enforcement may be required to achieve full impact.

Individual approaches through services

Some interventions taken up at the individual level – such as support for behaviour change, therapies, treatments and rehabilitation – can improve individual risk of premature mortality significantly, in some cases by 30–40%. The challenge is to achieve enough of those individual successes that they add up to percentage change at the population level. This will be achieved only if services take into account issues of system and scale to enable this to happen, and work to address population-level outcomes as well as those for individual service users.

Improvements in health and wellbeing will require some reorientation of health and other services to take a more holistic view of individual circumstances. These should take account of any personal characteristics/subpopulation group status or socioeconomic status and focus on development of personal skills of staff and service users, thus promoting healthy choices and actions.

Community approaches

Individuals will only choose to use and benefit from certain behaviours and actions if those behaviours fit with the cultural and belief system of their own community. Communities can be based on place (neighbourhood, school, workplace), culture (ethnicity, faith) and others (disability, sexual orientation). Community development is one way of facilitating communities' awareness of the factors and forces that affect their wellbeing, health and quality of life.

Community engagement is often patchy, favouring those communities that already have leadership, organisation and some resources. Instead, it needs to be systematic in bringing top–down and bottom–up priorities together into effective action plans. The aim should be to strengthen community action by creating more supportive environments for health improvement and developing the knowledge and skills of community members.

Service links into communities can be superficial, of poor quality, unsystematic and based on low levels of understanding. Connectivity between services can be disorganised and confusing. Use of the voluntary, community and faith sectors as a bridge between services and community-based structures needs to be systematic and based on need rather than supply. Effective commissioning is key to realising these objectives.

A holistic approach to commissioning: the 'Christmas tree' diagnostic

Substantial progress can be achieved in making an impact in the short, medium and long term in relation to inequalities in mortality and life expectancy through a focus on existing services. Because of this, extra attention is given here to extracting maximum benefit from delivery of interventions for which there is strong evidence base of effectiveness. In addition, there is a deliberate emphasis wherever possible on improving access to services at a scale that will bring about a population-level improvement in mortality and life expectancy within a 2–3-year period.

The detail is illustrated in the following diagram of commissioning services to best population-level outcomes, otherwise known as the 'Christmas tree' diagnostic, with an accompanying description of its component principles. The framework balances two sets of factors that determine whether optimal outcome can be achieved at the population level from a given set of personal health interventions (see Figure 7.4).

The right hand side of the diagram (1 to 5) – a challenge to providers – links the factors that will influence health *service* outcomes: that is, how can we construct the most effective service? However, optimal outcomes *at the population level* will not be obtained without combining this service focus with the other side.

The left hand side of the diagram (6 to 10) – a population focus – identifies those factors that determine whether a community makes best use of the service provided; for example, whether the benefits of personalised improvements to services are having a systematic impact on reducing health inequalities at the population level.

The balance between the two sides of the diagram is critical in determining what outcomes are secured, and designing an effective balance is the commissioning challenge: aiming for equality of

Figure 7.4: The 'Christmas tree'

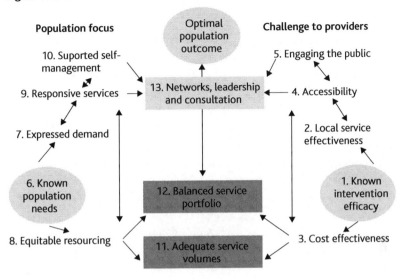

outcome, not just equality of access to service provision and support, is a significant and crucial challenge for commissioners. The Christmas tree diagnostic is a tool which can help them achieve a balance appropriate to their local circumstances. The right side of the diagram enables commissioners to identify the best services available for their population. The left side encourages them to consider how what is commissioned and delivered best meets the needs of all people in the local population. Attention to both sides of the diagram will help to make sure that all services are effective and engaged with, and used by all of the diverse communities in the area they serve.

The central elements of the diagram are concerned to ensure that, when the most effective services/interventions are identified that are fully acceptable, accessible and effective in terms of take-up and compliance, there is adequate capacity to meet the need. Effective leadership and networks are needed to ensure that all of these elements are being kept under review and to encourage continuous improvement and equality of morbidity and mortality outcomes.

Practical illustrations

The next section draws on some of the effective practice identified by HINST to illustrate each of the component parts of the Christmas tree model.

Efficacy

There is a well-established and strong evidence base in areas such as coronary heart disease, CVD and diabetes, which makes the case for those interventions that can be effective in reducing mortality. HINST commissioned modelling of a number of these to demonstrate the potential impact of the most effective of these interventions, and the tangible impact that systematic and scaled applications could have on mortality rates at the population level in a short timescale. The model was applied to all Spearheads to show the potential impact of evidence-based interventions. These were used by HINST as the basis of recommendations for evidence-based strategies during Spearhead visits.

Blackburn with Darwen Council/PCT, for example, addressed its variance from the inequalities target and used a systematic approach to quantify the impact of different, costed interventions on mortality, using the HINST evidence base. It produced a costed, evidence-based strategy that was adopted by the primary care trust (PCT) and local authority, based on HINST calculations of the numbers needed to be treated to postpone the death of a given number of people, using a tested set of interventions (see Figure 7.5).

Figure 7.5: Planning to reduce health inequalities through effective interventions – potential impact of evidence-based interventions on reducing mortality numbers (Blackburn with Darwen)

Intervention	Deaths postponed	Treatment population	NNT to postpone one death
Secondary prevention following CVD event (Four treatments: beta blocker, aspirin, ACE inhibitor, statin)			
Currently untreated: CVD deaths averted	20	926	45
Currently partially treated: CVD deaths averted	39	6,001	154
Additional treatment for hypertensives			
Additional hypertensive therapy	39	22,762	406
Statin treatment for hypertensives with high CVD risk	18		
Treatment for heart attack			
Primary angioplasty (PCI) for heart attack	2	227	107
Warfarin for atrial fibrillation >65 years			
Stroke deaths averted	10	352	37
Improving diabetes management			
Reducing blood sugars (HbA1c) over 7.5 by one unit	8	1,795	231
Treating CVD risk among COPD patients			
Statins for eligible mild and moderate COPD patients	24	964	40
Total	159	-	-

NNT = number needed to treat to postpone one death

Effectiveness

Once the evidence base is established, the impact of its application can still vary considerably, from place to place and even from clinician to clinician within a general practitioner (GP) practice, for example. HINST placed heavy emphasis on reducing local variation in primary care performance. It was possible to use the Quality and Outcomes Framework (QOF), collected as part of the GP contact, to identify significant variation and drive change. Figure 7.6 illustrates the difference between an area where there was unmanaged variation and, in contrast, the performance of Wakefield PCT. Here, GPs and primary care, supported by the PCT CVD team, were able to bring the performance of all practices up to the level of the best.

Cost-effectiveness

It is important that interventions intended to produce population-level impact can be cost-effective, so that they can be deployed at sufficient scale. HINST encountered examples where large gains could be achieved by improving the efficiency of current spending on such interventions. For example, Rotherham PCT illustrated the relationship between the average expenditure per patient with diabetes and their clinical outcomes, such as their level of blood sugar control (see Figure 7.7).

This diagram illustrates that there was no statistical relationship between the level of spend and outcome. The PCT was able to analyse the different prescribing patterns of GPs with high costs and poor outcomes, compared to the more cost-effective prescribing of those with low costs and good outcomes. The less cost-effective practices were then supported to improve their approach to prescribing to achieve a population health gain, while at the same time reducing costs.

Accessibility

Bringing services that deliver cost-effective interventions as close to the target population in need as possible is an important way of reducing barriers to access. In delivering its smoking cessation support programme, Knowsley PCT was providing the service through four centres across the district. The uptake was not sufficient to meet the PCT's 'quit target' or to achieve their ambition to reduce significantly the prevalence of smoking, and its impact on mortality. They therefore changed their strategic approach in order to achieve a

Figure 7.6: QOF data and 'unmanaged' and 'managed' variation in blood pressure (BP) reading

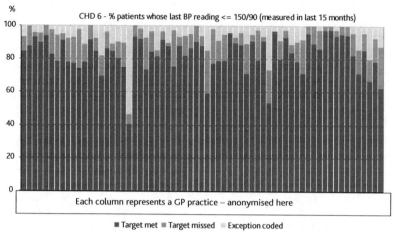

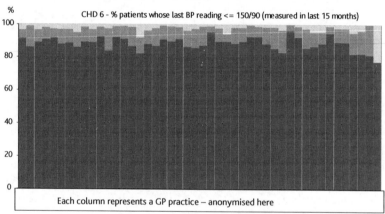

major amplification of the number of points from which services could be accessed. Eventually, services were delivered through 50, mainly community, venues. They were justifiably able to use the slogan 'Help is just around the corner'.

The Knowsley campaign generated a 154% increase in numbers coming into the service in the first six months, and almost a 200% increase in smoking quitters.

Figure 7.7: Rotherham prescribing costs per diabetic patient (April 2006 – March 2007) vs. percentage of diabetic patients whose HbA1C has been 7.4 or less in the last 15 months (April 2006 – March 2007)

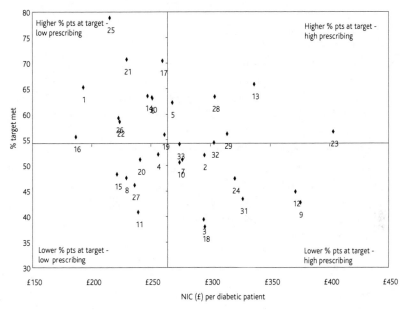

Engagement

Engagement with users and potential users of services is critical to ensure that services meet the needs of patients rather than those of the delivery systems themselves. As part of this it is important to connect with those who failed to take up an offer of service, or dropped out of a service programme, rather than those who are easier to access or more compliant with the current service design.

Four phases of rehabilitation are recommended following a heart attack or heart surgery. In most systems patients can be lost at various points along the pathway. In Sunderland they had managed to reduce this attrition substantially through the first three stages of the process, but then recorded a dramatic fall-off before stage IV. This stage was the point at which the venue for rehabilitation moved from a health care setting into leisure services. An exercise of tracking patients who failed to attend at stage IV uncovered real concerns that they were worried about leaving the perceived safety and care of professional health care staff to transfer to non-medical leisure services staff.

This was addressed by bringing the leisure services staff into the programme at stage III. This enabled patients to get to know leisure services staff and build confidence in their ability to maintain levels of care before the transition. Attendance for stage IV of the programme increased significantly.

Population needs assessment

Population health programmes require interventions to be delivered in complex environments. Elements in these environments will influence the success or otherwise of delivery. HINST found that the public health evidence base has not paid sufficient attention to defining the context of delivery.

Public health teams in South Yorkshire worked with Sheffield Hallam University on cluster analysis of previously defined 'natural neighbourhoods'. By modelling a range of measures available at the neighbourhood level the team was able to identify 20 cluster types, each of which was distinct in its characteristics from the others (see Figure 7.8).

Figure 7.8: South Yorkshire neighbourhood clustering

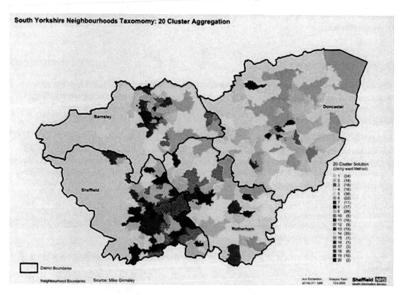

The importance of this was that neighbourhoods of the same cluster type/colour had more similar characteristics to each other than they had to their geographical neighbours. It followed that interventions that were effective in a neighbourhood of one cluster type could be tried in other neighbourhoods that shared that cluster type. This could then be used as the basis of planning interventions

Seven neighbourhood cluster types were identified:

- older large estates
- new estates
- rural and small towns
- ex-coalfields communities
- mixed young families
- established non-Caucasian ethnic
- mobile young.

It can be seen that the basis of deprivation in an ex-mining community is likely to be different from that of a neighbourhood largely comprised of ethnic minorities or an inner-city estate.

Expressed demand

Figure 7.9 gives a stark representation of the problems that HINST came to describe as 'the missing thousands'. The map of the City of Birmingham on the left gives the number of patients registered with their GP as having coronary heart disease. The map on the right shows the standardised mortality rate due to heart disease. The two together demonstrate the complete mismatch between the level of expressed demand registered with GPs and the actual level of need.

Even if the quality of services is good, if patients drop out and do not connect with them appropriately they will have little impact. The best example HINST saw of a systematic initiative to address this problem

Figure 7.9: 'The missing thousands'

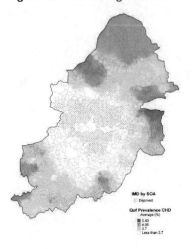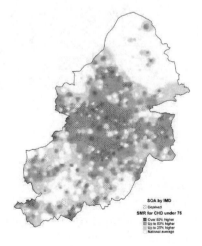

was at Bolton. A programme was commissioned in 2009 to screen as high a proportion of the eligible population as possible for heart disease risk, raised blood pressure and diabetes – the 'Big Bolton Healthcheck'. Although based in primary care, it recruited support from across the local community, including health and social care frontline services, the voluntary sector and commercial pharmacies. The local press backed the campaign with regular articles and updates to raise awareness. The programme became a significant community-wide event.

As a result, within the year 85% of the eligible population was screened. This was balanced across all districts of the borough, including the most deprived areas. Dramatically, some 800 people were newly diagnosed with diabetes and some 1,200 with renal disease. This previously undiscovered reservoir of unmet need could then be registered, thereby enabling GPs to provide treatment systematically for people who were previously missing out.

The issue of the 'missing thousands' is one that was found to be almost universal across all the Spearhead areas visited. Hence, HINST began to represent the scale of this problem using data shown in Figure 7.10. This diagram builds on the chart showing the intermediate outcomes of health care in Figure 7.6 earlier, but in addition, the lightest grey section of each bar provides an estimate of how many patients with each condition are currently missing from the relevant practice disease register.

Figure 7.10: Identifying the proportion of untreated patients

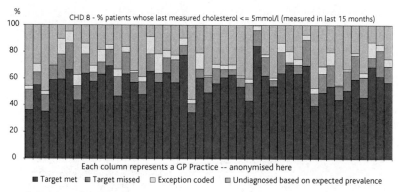

Equitable resourcing

In addressing health inequalities it is important to tailor the resources available to meet differential needs across the population. However, the focus needs to be less on equality of inputs, according to need, and more on the resource necessary to achieve equitable outcomes. HINST found that in most areas a proportion of the population containing the most vulnerable people living in the most chaotic environments needed a disproportionate amount of resources to achieve the same sort of outcomes that were possible for others.

An important example was found in the QOF incentive scheme, which rewards achievement of only up to 70% of target blood pressure in people with coronary heart disease. The problem from a health inequalities perspective is that many of the most vulnerable people are likely to remain in the unmanaged remaining 30%. This was addressed, again in Bolton, by recasting the incentive scheme to reward effort on an exponential scale that heavily incentivised reaching successful outcomes with people who were hard to reach (see Figure 7.11). An enhanced payment system was introduced to maximise CHD assessments by GPs. It can be seen from Figure 7.11 if a Practice achieves only 50% coverage they are paid £2 per patient and if it achieves 90% it is paid £9 for every single patient, recognising the exponential effort and resource that is needed to include hard to reach patients.

Figure 7.11: Logarithmic incentivisation

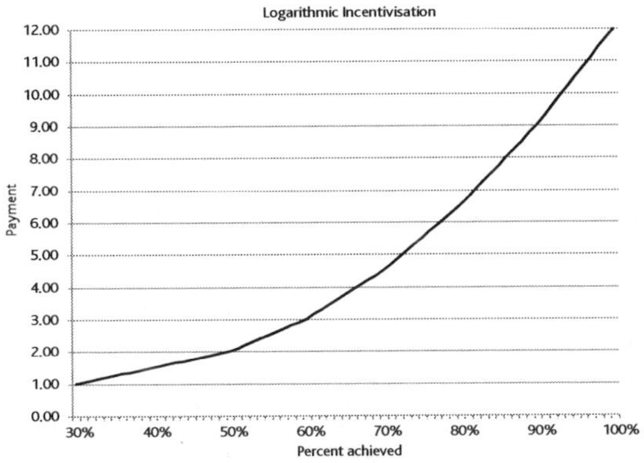

Achievement	Reward
30%	£ 1.00
40%	£ 1.50
50%	£ 2.00
60%	£ 3.00
70%	£ 4.50
80%	£ 6.50
90%	£ 9.00
100%	£12.00

Responsive services

When patients do come forward and present to services it is critical that their early contacts are positive and engaging, to ensure that the opportunity is taken to diagnose their illness at a point when it is accessible to treatment. In Doncaster, where lung cancer mortality among men is a significant problem, it was found that most patients were presenting too late for effective treatment. Part of the solution was to raise the knowledge and expectations of the population, to encourage people to come forward (increasing 'expressed demand'). However, Suckling (2010) has suggested that patients often did not think it worthwhile to come forward as their GP, when faced with new chest symptoms, would just prescribe antibiotics without carrying out further tests. A second study showed that because a large proportion of these patients were smokers and had a chronic cough the GPs rarely referred them for X-ray (which could potentially have detected cancers at an earlier, treatable stage), believing that it would be unlikely to be helpful in many cases.

A systematic programme was launched to raise the awareness of GPs of the National Institute for Health and Care Excellence (NICE) guidance on the indicators of early lung cancer and the criteria for referral for chest X-rays, which had been recently published. This led to a significant change in practice. The hospital radiology department was included in the initiative so that it was able to manage the increased number of referrals resulting from a change in the threshold of referral.

The increase in patient self-referral, combined with more responsive frontline services, resulted in a dramatic shift in the percentage of patients potentially eligible for surgical treatment from 11% to 19% (see Figure 7.12).

Figure 7.12: Comparison of stage of diagnosis with previous year

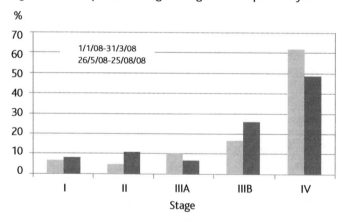

Supported self-care

Once diagnosis is made and care packages are prescribed, patients need to manage their use of the interventions themselves for much of the time. If not used appropriately, outcomes will be limited, however potentially effective the planned treatment was. When a range of medications remains untaken 'in the bathroom cabinet', for example, the predicted outcomes will not be achieved. Preparing patients and supporting them to self-manage medication and other treatment should be an important part of the care plan. However, the HINST experience is that this was often not the case.

A significant example was provided by a major teaching hospital, which has received accolades for the quality of its self-management training for patients diagnosed with type 2 diabetes. Patients provided very positive feedback and the service was held up as an exemplar for others on how to run such a service in innovative ways. However, further review showed that the capacity of the programme was just over 200 patients per year, while the number of newly diagnosed diabetics was over 1,000 per year. This was reflected in the population outcomes, when the proportion of patients whose blood sugar levels were within target levels was shown to be well below 50%.

From a population perspective it would be important to provide effective self-management training at a scale to make it available to the majority of the population, rather than providing excellent training to a relatively small minority.

Adequate service volumes

HINST predicted, and subsequently observed, that for action to make an impact at the population level it needs to be systematic and resourced at the right scale. It is important that adequate service volumes are commissioned to aim for, and ensure, acceptable access times. 'Process mapping' can assist in the commissioning process here. For example, have all partners involved in delivering diabetes care carried out a process mapping exercise to help identify areas where there are inefficiencies, lack of resources or duplication? Have the outcomes been acted upon? A second approach to developing adequate service volumes is related to 'walking the patient journey'. For example, have techniques been used to gain a real picture of the issues and problems for patients as they move through the care pathway (for example, patient shadowing, tracing the patient's journey through a study of records)?[47]

Balanced service portfolio

Patient pathways of care and the more complex array of support required, for example in the management of long term conditions, can sometimes be baffling for patients. There may be gaps in the pathway or barriers to parts of their care programme. It is clear that patients in the most complex and vulnerable situations will be among the first to fall at any of these hurdles. This was found to be the case by the Wakefield Diabetes Care Service.

When the capabilities of GPs were reviewed across the patch they found that there was great variability on the level of knowledge and skills relating to diabetes care. They were able to assess these and grade the capability of each practice on a multi-point scale.[48] In this respect, a Level 1 practice would be limited to a smaller number of capabilities than a Level 4 (these capabilities are outlined in Figure 7.13). This meant that, if all patients were to receive their required level of service, a variable level of compensatory input was necessary from secondary care specialists (see Figure 7.13).

However, assessment suggested that services did not match exactly and that patients would 'fall through the gaps' (see Figure 7.14).

In an agreed programme the secondary care clinicians came into primary care to provide a period of joint management of complex patients together with the patient's own GP. This raised skill levels across primary care demonstrably, so that after two years no practices were classified within the lower levels of capability 1–2 (see Figure 7.15).

The resulting agreements on joint working and increased clinical confidence in primary care led to significant improvements in clinical outcomes for patients and greater levels of professional satisfaction among the practitioners

Networks, leadership and coordination

Networks provide a framework for identifying and sharing effective practice. HINST worked with the Merseyside and Cheshire Cancer Network to scope the ways that cancer networks could have an impact on health inequalities. This Network was chosen because it had a well-developed strategy for reducing heath inequalities, with a range of effective, practical tools.[49]

The steps identified in the development of a coherent strategy to reduce mortality from cancers were as follows.

- Develop a clear vision shared across the Network about what the future could look like – taking everybody forward together.
- Develop a strategic plan which prioritises areas of greatest need where change is possible – tackling shared problems together.
- This needs to be based on best evidence and regional experience – taking into account cost-effectiveness.

Figure 7.13: Wakefield classification of levels of specialist and generalist clinical skills in treating diabetes

	Prevention Identification Impaired Glucose Tolerance/ Impaired Fasting Glucose Diet controlled Type 2 diabetes	Type 2 on tablets Annual review	Management of patients stablised on insulin Annual review Type 1 and Type 2 diabetes	Initiation of insulin Problem patients Unstable diabetes Annual review Type 1 and Type 2 diabetes	Gestational diabetes Pre-conception care Children and adolescents In-patient hospital care Complex complications Insulin pump Carbohydrate counting DAFNE
Practice Level 1					
Practice Level 2					
Practice Level 3					
Practice Level 4					

Primary care

Specialist care

Figure 7.14: Mismatch in specialist and generalist provision leading to patients falling between the gaps

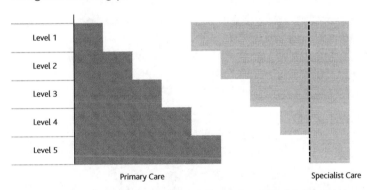

Level 1
Level 2
Level 3
Level 4
Level 5

Primary Care   Specialist Care

Figure 7.15: Structured collaboration leading to raised skill levels in primary care

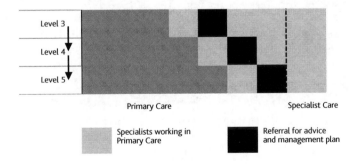

Level 3
Level 4
Level 5

Primary Care   Specialist Care

Specialists working in Primary Care

Referral for advice and management plan

- The strategic plan also needs to include a transparent process for reviewing progress and feeding back to the constituent members of the Network – including the emerging commissioners.

Cancer networks have the potential to establish a direct link between poor outcomes at the population level and conventional service improvement approaches by:

- identifying anomalies in outcomes (particularly when incidence is average);
- producing explanations for them;
- recommending interventions of sufficient scale to have a quantified impact on mortality;
- targeting the patient pathways that result in poor outcomes;
- engaging all stakeholders (patients and potential service users, clinical groups, primary care, commissioning and public health) involved along the pathway in a comprehensive action plan;carrying out a series of major network locality change management events to ensure translation of needs into action and sharing of good practice;
- assisting in obtaining finance for the key actions.

The variations that exist are startling – Figure 7.16 shows an example of the route that patients took to reach the specialist treatment they needed, by GP practice. Networks, working with NHS England and clinical support units, are ideally placed to explore why some practices are able to manage patient referral – and may have effective practice

Figure 7.16: Variation in the rate of managed presentation by general practice

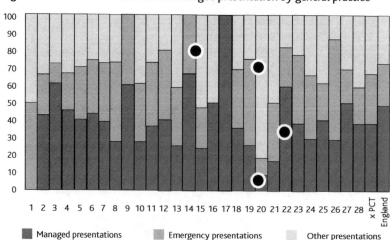

to share with those that are less able. HINST recommends that cancer networks facilitate the development of the framework for pathways of care, in the first instance for the cancers that cause most deaths – lung, breast and colorectal. A generic approach common to other cancers may then emerge with some key characteristics:

- the work could link to work getting underway through National Cancer Action Team (NCAT) on the Map of Medicine – a library of evidence based practice for clinicians. For interest see: http://mapofmedicine.com/about;
- the ambition should be on a 'spine' for the whole pathway, from patient awareness and decision to present with symptoms/signs, through reception and management in primary care, to referral and engagement by specialist services, living with cancer, and finally end–of–life care; the emphasis would be determining fixed elements of process, but allowing room for substantial variation by locality;
- the pathway should define the 'what', leaving the 'how', where appropriate, to local ownership and innovation.

These underlying principles apply to most clinical networks, which are going to be in a critical position in having both an overview vantage point to be able to identify local effective action and those areas where there are issues at one of the other 13 points of the Christmas tree diagnostic.[45]

The new environment: requirements for delivering population-level change through the new policy structure

Localism is the foundation of the public health system introduced in 2013, and progress against health inequalities will require strong local partnerships, led by local government, to address the 'wicked' public health problems that sustain health inequalities. The scale of these problems is such that they will require industrial-scale interventions, rather than piecemeal initiatives. Many partnerships have achieved great success, but many have not and will struggle to do this without support, given the fiscal environment of the austerity current measures. The new public health system will not have a centralised performance-management system and Public Health England (PHE), in its role supporting transformational change locally, will have to build and adapt approaches that enable partnerships to choose their own priorities, and come together and review their collective endeavours against international evidence and the successes of others elsewhere.

The approach of HINST is consistent with these principles. Ten aspects of the HINST approach are now highlighted that may be of use to PHE and others working to support local partnerships in the new environment. Applying the evidence-based learning from HINST to the emerging environment, it is possible to identify the following ways in which the new public health system could be developed to address health inequalities.

Achieving percentage change at the population level for any selected outcome means taking account, particularly, of system, scale and sustainability of evidence-based interventions. Delivering within the new policy structures may require the following issues to be addressed.

Governance: who is running the show?

If health and wellbeing boards (HWBs) are to deliver on the health and wellbeing strategy they will need to establish strong governance arrangements. As statutory bodies they will be held accountable for their own delivery by local residents/electorate, by constituent bodies such as the cabinet and clinical commissioning groups (CCGs), and through some national agreements – for example, PHE health premium plans. Style will include decisions as to whether they constitute a 'strategic forum' for collective action, or whether they develop a performance-management function with which to deliver integrated programmes

Joint strategic needs assessments

Joint strategic needs assessments (JSNAs) should start from a systematic balanced, non-judgemental overview of health, social care and wellbeing issues, followed by a more detailed drilling down on emerging important issues. They should combine a top-down more quantitative analysis with bottom-up more qualitative inputs from communities, service users and frontline staff. Each prioritised topic should be broken down into meaningful causative elements that might be addressed. JSNAs should not stop at describing problems, but should proceed to highlighting the 'so-what': possible consequences and potential actions. Ideally, needs-based assessment could be balanced with an assessment of assets. A JSNA should be a process, not a document (or website). Findings should ideally move from dry analysis to 'marketing' the findings to a range of audiences (elected members; local authority officers; GP commissioners; HealthWatch and the public).

Priority setting: how does it really work?

Priority setting will usually involve a consultation process and debate, for which officers will be involved in making cases and options appraisal. This is the part of the process where corporate ownership of issues is won or lost, reaching for the hearts and minds of members. The 'anatomy' of a decision is said to be in three parts: evidence, ethics and politics. Case makers will need to take into account all three elements, not just rely on evidence. Debate in a local authority setting is more often emotive rather than scientific/technical. A good example of working with this is referring to 'the number of men or women dying' for comparative purposes, rather than 'differences in mortality rates projected for each sex'.

Setting targets: locally relevant and meaningful

In setting targets, choosing testing but achievable benchmarks for change (for example, levels achieved by 'best in class' for Office for National Statistics (ONS) peer authority cluster) and setting 'SMART' (specific, measurable, achievable, realistic, timely) objectives, with numbers where possible, are both important issues to address. Where relevant and it makes sense, national outcomes frameworks and indicators should be taken into account. Distributional factors need to be considered, via use needs assessments and equity audits to establish the need for graded or targeted responses within an area. Comparison should be meaningful to local stakeholders. Offers of support to local partnerships need to combine those areas the local partnerships want to work on with those identified as having the biggest potential impact on life expectancy. The two may be different. In the new public health system there is no mandate for centrally defined, hierarchically managed targets. Support from regional and national bodies will have to incorporate locally defined priorities.

Whole system approach

Complex programmes for population-level change will not all be delivered through conventional services, and may well involve all three points of the population-level intervention triangle:

- population-level interventions (healthy public policy, legislation, regulation, licensing);

- systematic and scaled intervention through primary, community and hospital based services; wraparound social care; third sector support);
- systematic community engagement.

The triangle (see Figure 7.3 earlier) could provide a useful framework and specification for the population–based working of the HWB.

Select interventions: strongly evidence-based

The evidence base should be reviewed to establish interventions that could make a substantial contribution to the target. This should capitalise on evidence sources across the sectors involved (including health, social care, housing and community engagement). The size of the potential contribution for each proposed intervention should be modelled or estimated. The scope for improvement utilising the proposed interventions should explored, and consideration given to what systems will be necessary to deliver the scale of intervention necessary.

Develop a business plan: economic case for change

With systems, scale and timescale established, cost and potential return on investment should be modelled to make a viable business case. It may often be a case for changing focus of existing programmes, rather than starting a whole new programme afresh. In standing up to competition for resources, the persuasiveness of the case can be supported through a well-managed and widely owned prioritisation process (see above). Finally, the business plan will need to take into account the different business planning models and cycles of the component sectors and organisations.

Programme planning: who is responsible?

The components of strategy contributing to a priority outcome should be brought together in a defined cohesive programme. Different components will often be delivered by different organisations. However, it would be preferable if there were a single empowered lead answerable to the local Health and Wellbeing Board for each prioritised health and wellbeing strategy outcome.

Information governance: sharing intelligence

The health and wellbeing strategy would benefit from being accompanied by a number of support strategies, in particular:

• an information governance strategy exploring and facilitating the flows of data and information around the system, necessary for delivery of the strategy and its programmes;a communication strategy, marketing information through partner organisations and the wider public, about the JSNA findings, and the health and wellbeing strategy and its progress.

Maximise impact: minimise inequalities

In relation to delivery through services, there are many factors that influence whether an intervention, or group of interventions, has the optimal impact at the population level. HINST used a checklist of 13 factors, pulled together as the Christmas tree diagnostic (see Figure 7.4 earlier). Many of the 13 factors in this diagnostic are often neglected in designing and running programmes, resulting in patchy delivery, well below the programme potential. HWBs could provide a milieu, through connectivity between services and with community infrastructures, to develop population connectivity with services (left hand side of the diagnostic) which they have previously not been utilising appropriately.

Concluding discussion: capitalising on the hinst model

In the new policy context there has been a move away from nationally defined targets, towards localism. Desired outcomes of policy are to be locally defined and owned, with encouragement to set some of them within a set of national outcomes frameworks. Accountability will be more to resident populations and their elected representatives, rather than through performance management to national government. However, such accountability will still need to be demonstrable, with significant change at the (local) population level. It will also, pragmatically, need to demonstrate measureable progress within the short timescale between local elections. Localism offers the benefits of local ownership, relevance and accountability. However, among the possible dis-benefits of such a 'devolved' structure can be isolationism, patchiness and variability.

The model of support offered by the national support teams, including HINST, could be particularly relevant in this new environment, for a number of key reasons.

- The teams worked separately from any performance-management structures, bringing an external perspective and an approach that was 'high challenge; high support'.
- The teams were linked *to* 'the Centre' (the Department of Health), bringing empowerment and credibility, but not *of* the Centre and feeding back judgements.
- The local area leadership was designated as the 'client', with feedback and recommendations directed to them only, and onward distribution by them at their discretion.
- Once trust in these principles was established, it was possible to get more honest, and less sanitised, inputs through interviews and workshops.
- Using the structured approaches to assessment and inquiry, the teams were able to identify good practice as well as common gaps and barriers to progress. These could then be disseminated:
  - horizontally, to other local areas by matching local specific needs to relevant good practice;
  - vertically, assimilating frontline experience and feeding back to the Centre in aggregated and anonymised form, to influence policy.
- Beyond assessment and recommendation, teams were able to use the principles of change management to influence and 'unblock' local politics – for example, by introducing external perspectives and benchmarks to local leaders and opinion formers.

In the context of this book the work of HINST offers an insight into the issues encountered in developing an applied approach to health inequalities. The HINST experience suggests that it is possible to narrow gaps in health outcomes based on policy action. The Team did not have the remit to test the alternative premise, set out in chapter one above, that health inequalities are a wicked problem that require change in the structure of the economy and society. However HINST came to believe that the systematic approach they developed could impact on the range of components that constitute the complex problem that is health inequalities.

EIGHT

Qualitative comparative analysis case study

Introduction

This chapter draws on case study research using the qualitative comparative analysis (QCA) methodology to develop understandings of what works in addressing complex policy problems such as health inequalities. The research (conducted by Blackman, Byrne and J. Wistow between 2007 and 2010[50]) sought to investigate why there were significant differences across the 70 Spearhead local authority areas in England in the extent to which they made progress towards their 2010 health inequality targets. In so doing, the research developed a whole system approach to understanding health inequalities (as outlined in Chapter Three) that accounted for the socially structured nature of health and the importance of locally determined actions and ways of working to address health inequalities. By adopting a holistic perspective for a QCA, each individual case is considered as a combination of properties – a specific 'whole' that should not be lost or obscured in the analysis (Berg-Schlosser et al, 2009). Consequently, complex cases – such as Spearhead areas – can be compared systematically by transforming the cases into configurations of conditions and analysing how these combine, with a given outcome of interest (Rihoux and Ragin, 2009). Case studies can provide inferential leverage on complex causation by utilising within-case analysis or cross-case comparison (Bennett and Elman, 2006). Fiss (2009) argues that case study approaches benefit from employing set-theoretic methods such as QCA that fit with the assumptions of complex causal interdependencies. Outcomes can be treated as the consequences of interactions between multiple conditions, and there is recognition that the same outcome may be generated by different configurations of conditions.

This chapter focuses on the results of our analysis and introduces a methodology that can identify interactions between context and agency (in this example, using the local authorities as cases) in progress towards narrowing health inequality gaps. It consists of six sections. First, a brief overview of the background to the research project is provided. The following section introduces the methodology used for the study. This is followed by sections on the results of the study and a discussion of the findings. The next section is concerned with implications for policy and practice that arise from the study. The final section provides some reflections on the overall learning and common threads arising from the study.

Background to the study

The study was concerned with understanding reported variations in the success of actions to reduce health inequalities in English local authorities with high deprivation and health needs (the so-called 'Spearhead' areas). It focused, therefore, on a key issue identified in both policy and research: the extent and nature of differences in practice and outcomes relating to health inequalities. For example, the Department of Health (DH)'s 2007 status report *Tackling health inequalities: Programme for action* stated that the 2010 target was achievable if local action was focused, evidence-based and managed through effective systems for accountability and performance management (DH, 2007d). However, a great deal of local variation in progress within, and between, Spearheads was also identified. Even so, the report stated that if the positive trend for life expectancy in some Spearhead areas was replicated in all, the target would be more than met within the specified period.

Studies by Tunstall et al (2007) and Walsh et al (2007) have also identified variations in progress with narrowing health inequalities among areas with similar levels of economic deprivation. Tunstall et al note that 'if some areas can resist the translation of economic adversity into higher mortality, other areas can learn from their policies and approaches' (2007: 342). The main objective of the study discussed in this chapter was to identify how such learning can occur on the basis of understanding the features of local areas in which health inequalities had been narrowing. Over the course of the research a series of local conditions[51] were identified that were considered likely to assist in narrowing the differences between these outcomes. Such conditions are discussed fully in Chapter Three and included, for example, how well partnerships were working and whether best practices likely to have a high impact on improving health in the most disadvantaged communities were, in fact, in place. Once these conditions were identified, local stakeholders were asked to assess[52] their Spearhead area against them. Assessments for each area, along with contextual information such as the level of deprivation, were analysed using the qualitative comparative analysis computer package fsQCA that identifies how conditions combine together to associate with outcomes. The project explored what combinations of practice and context were associated with most progress.

The outcome measures we used were local trends in premature mortality (deaths under 75 years of age) from cancers and circulatory diseases, together with teenage conception rates for each Spearhead area, all compared to the national trend (England average). To explore associations between the conditions in the Spearhead areas and the trajectory of change in the extent of health inequalities in each area, we used 2004 outcome data for our baseline and 2007 data for our final data point, the most recent available data at the time of the study. Our analysis was, therefore, looking for quite short-term effects on the inequality gap, based on assessments of local conditions made in 2005 (see Blackman et al, 2011b). The teenage conception analysis was updated for a paper by Blackman et al (2013) and the 2005 baseline data was compared with the 2009 difference between each area's local teenage conception rate and the national rate. Our assessments of outcome trends were based on a combination of approaches which enabled us to judge whether an area was narrowing or not narrowing its gap with the national rate, including visualisation of projections and a calculation of the absolute and relative differences between 2004 and 2007[53] (the Spearhead area compared to the England average).

Methodology

QCA can be regarded as a methodological response to the increasing complexity of the societies in which we live. As discussed in Part One of the book, quantitative approaches to causality in social science have conventionally had in common a focus on the relation between supposedly independent (predictive and/or causal) variables and a dependent outcome variable. Attempts are made to locate the independent average net effect of one variable on another, while controlling for the effects of other independent variables. Causal homogeneity – the idea that causes act in the same way across all cases – is often assumed, and it is usually only in particular specialist fields that the possibility of causal heterogeneity is addressed (see, for example, Clark et al, 2006; Morgan and Winship, 2007; Goldstein, 2010). Crucially, however, the central idea is still one of isolating the independent effect of one variable on an outcome while controlling for others.

Our research was based on a very different premise: that causes act in combination. We used QCA to capture this causal complexity. To quote Buijs et al:

> ...this allows for the specification of complex and contingent causes ... which are however not unique, but may in fact be shared across a number of cases. This allows the researcher to develop knowledge beyond the detailed ideographic description of unique instances. (2009: 45)

QCA is an innovative approach in public health research but is more established in other fields, including organisational research (Ragin, 1987; 2000; 2006a; 2006b; 2008; Cooper, 2005; Longest and Vaisey, 2008; Fiss, 2009; Glaesser et al, 2009a, 2009b; Grofman and Schneider, 2009; Olsen and Nomura, 2009; Rihoux and Ragin, 2009). It uses an approach to elucidating causality that investigates an outcome (for example, whether a locality is closing its health inequalities gap with the national average) as the product of how conditions combine together rather than have independent effects. As noted in Chapter Two, it is possible to consider health inequality targets as being addressed by a local system, and outcomes from this system can be seen as a reflection of the purposeful design of services, the nature of interactions between agents, and contextual conditions (Wrede et al, 2006).

In Chapter Three it is argued that variable-based methods such as regression techniques seek to estimate the average effect of particular independent variables, which may or may not be reflected in any individual case, and that QCA, instead, seeks to explain why specific cases have particular outcomes. QCA is fundamentally a qualitative method. Ragin (1987; 2000; 2008) has built the method on insights from the qualitative case study, especially how conditions depend on the state of other conditions characterising the case. QCA allocates cases to sets, which are shared configurations of conditions. By including causal conditions with an outcome condition, possible causal pathways can be identified. The method does not involve specifying a single causal model that best fits the data, but instead involves determining the number and character of the different causal models that exist among the cases (Berg–Schlosser et al, 2009; Byrne, 2009). To quote Ragin:

> An especially useful feature of QCA is its capacity for analyzing complex causation, defined as a situation in which an outcome may follow from several different combinations of causal conditions, that is, from different causal 'recipes' ...

> By examining the fate of cases with different configurations of causally relevant conditions, it is possible, using QCA, to identify the decisive recipes and thereby unravel causal complexity. (2008: 23)

QCA enables causal arguments to be made by creating a very close correspondence between theory and data analysis, analysing evidence in ways that directly address theoretical arguments about what matters to achieve some outcome. This makes QCA especially appropriate for policy research; the process of defining conditions is then also a process of identifying either manipulable or contextual conditions necessary for producing a policy outcome. Chapter Three (in the section on conditions in whole systems) provided a detailed summary of conditions that can be considered to have potential impacts on health inequalities within local authority areas. This whole system approach created a very long list of conditions for the QCA study. In the section of Chapter Three entitled 'Causation is binary even if it is complex', we describe our approach to reducing the number of conditions to a more manageable number for the QCA.

A central concern of QCA is to explore whether individual conditions or different combinations of them are either necessary or sufficient to produce an outcome. There are two principles to follow in this respect.

- When a condition or particular configuration of conditions is *necessary* for an outcome, all instances of a given outcome should exhibit the same condition or configuration, although a different outcome may also occur.
- When a condition or configuration is *sufficient* for an outcome, all instances of the condition or configuration should be associated with the outcome, although the outcome could also occur with other conditions.

The specific QCA technique employed in this study has its roots in the earliest and most widely used application of the method, developed by Ragin and now known as 'crisp set' (csQCA). This uses binary data based on a condition being either *present* or *absent* (variables with values of 1 or 0, such as 'yes' or 'no'). It therefore relies on the dichotomisation of variables. Chapter Three outlines the rationale for dichotomising these for a csQCA. The data was coded for analysis using SPSS (the statistical package for the social sciences) and fsQCA. The fsQCA package works out combinations of conditions associated with given outcomes: in this case, whether or not health inequalities had been narrowing. What causal factors or conditions are included in the model is a matter of judgement based on the wider evidence base, theory and empirical analysis.

The provisional results of the study were circulated to all participating primary care trusts (PCTs) and subsequently discussed with participants at a series of workshops in September and October 2009. This ensured that the results were more firmly grounded in, and coloured by, practitioners' experiences and knowledge. Insights provided through the workshops have been incorporated into the commentary on the study results below.

Out of a total of 70 Spearhead areas, 34 completed at least one of the questionnaires. For cancers, 29 areas returned the questionnaire, with complete returns for 27 areas; for cardiovascular disease (CVD), 33 areas returned the questionnaire, with complete returns from 27 areas; and for teenage conceptions, 31 areas returned the questionnaires, with complete returns from 27 areas. A Mann-Whitney statistical test was conducted to establish whether there was any difference between the areas participating in the study and the non-responding Spearhead areas. The five factors used for determining Spearhead status (outlined in Chapters One and Eight) were employed for this test. For four[54] of these, no significant difference was found between the participating group and the other Spearhead areas.

Results

The results of the QCA study are provided in Tables 8.1 (cancers), 8.2 (CVD) and 8.3 (teenage conceptions). It is important to note that because there were a number of overlapping and contradictory configurations in the results it was only possible to develop dichotomised data tables and not 'truth tables'[55] (see Rihoux and Ragin, 2009). Given the intrinsic complexity of our subject matter, some anomalous results were to be expected. Nonetheless, we were able to use the data we collected to produce systematic comparisons of conditions with clear skews or associations towards either narrowing or not narrowing outcomes, using the set-theoretic and configurational approach of QCA to focus on *combinations* of conditions within the configurations. The exploratory use of QCA also employs contradictory configurations as a guide to further exploration of the data, and that is precisely what we did through revisiting the dataset and our dialogues with practitioners in the workshops.

Cancers[56]

The results of the cancers QCA are included in Table 8.1. This includes the configurations of conditions found to have strong relationships in combination with whether the cancers gap was narrowing or not. More detailed descriptions of these conditions are provided in Appendix B. Of the 27 Spearhead areas in this part of our analysis, 12 had a narrowing gap for cancers. One condition – 'championing' – was present in each of these 12 cases and was, therefore, identified as a necessary condition for this outcome. We then looked at what factors were combined with championing in the 12 areas where inequalities between local and national cancer outcomes had narrowed. We found that in nine cases championing was combined with higher spending on cancer. This configuration of conditions was considered a sufficient combination for narrowing, since there were no cases with this combination in which the gap was not narrowing. The second narrowing combination has seven cases in a combination of championing, basic workforce planning, less frequent monitoring and lower deprivation. There are two contradictory 'not narrowing' cases with this combination. The third narrowing combination is also sufficient and consists of championing and an aspirational organisational culture, combined with some surprising and apparently counter-intuitive conditions: a basic public health workforce, less frequent monitoring, higher deprivation and higher crime.

There are three combinations with an outcome of not narrowing the cancer gap. In the first, the surprising and counter–intuitive results for two of the narrowing combinations have their mirror images, together with a further surprising result regarding partnership working. This combination combines good or exemplary commissioning, good or exemplary strategic partnership working, a good or exemplary public health workforce and an aspirational organisational culture. With six cases and no contradictions, this configuration can be categorised as sufficient for the gap to not be narrowing. The second combination combines a comfortable or complacent organisational culture with higher crime, lower spending on cancer programmes, a lower performing PCT (based on a national exercise assessing PCT performance across all functions) and lower deprivation. This configuration (found in two of the not narrowing cases) also occurs for cases where cancer inequalities have failed to close. Finally, the third combination combines a comfortable or complacent organisational culture, higher crime, a basic public health workforce and less frequent monitoring. Four not narrowing cases are in the combination but also

Table 8.1: Conditions associated with a narrowing gap in cancers mortality (1=present; 0=absent)

	Area	Basic commissioning	Less than good strategic partnership working	Less than good public health workforce planning	Less frequent progress reviews	Champions	Aspirational	Lower IMD	Higher spend on cancers	Lower crime	3 star PCT
GAP NARROWING	1	1	No data	1	0	1	0	0	1	0	0
	2	1	1	1	1	1	1	1	1	0	1
	3	No data	1	1	1	1	1	1	1	1	1
	4	1	1	1	1	1	1	1	0	1	1
	5	0	1	1	1	1	1	1	1	1	0
	6	1	1	1	1	1	0	1	1	1	1
	7	1	1	1	1	1	0	1	0	1	1
	8	1	0	1	1	1	0	1	1	0	0
	9	1	1	1	1	1	1	0	1	0	0
	10	0	0	1	1	1	1	0	1	0	1
	11	1	0	1	1	1	1	0	0	0	0
	12	1	1	0	1	1	0	0	1	0	0
GAP NOT NARROWING	13	0	1	1	1	1	1	0	0	1	0
	14	1	1	1	1	1	0	1	0	1	1
	15	0	1	1	1	1	0	1	0	0	0
	16	0	0	0	0	0	1	0	1	0	0
	17	0	0	0	1	0	1	0	0	0	0
	18	0	0	0	0	0	1	1	1	0	1
	19	0	0	0	1	0	1	0	0	0	1
	20	0	0	0	1	1	1	1	0	0	0
	21	0	0	0	0	0	1	1	1	1	0
	22	0	0	1	1	0	0	0	0	0	0
	23	0	1	1	1	0	0	0	0	0	0
	24	0	1	1	1	0	0	1	1	0	1
	25	1	1	1	1	1	0	0	0	0	1
	26	1	1	1	No data	1	0	1	0	0	0
	27	0	0	1	0	0	1	1	1	0	0

Key:

Config 1 ☐   Config 2 ▨   Config 3 ▨   Config 4 ▨   Config 5 ☐   Config 6 ☐

one narrowing case, which makes this a contradictory configuration but one associated with not narrowing outcomes.

CVD

The different combinations of conditions associated with narrowing and not narrowing CVD outcomes are shown in Table 8.2. More detailed descriptions of these conditions are found in Appendix B. Neither necessary conditions nor sufficient combinations could be

Table 8.2: Conditions associated with a narrowing gap in CVD mortality (1=present; 0=absent)

	Area	Better than basic smoking cessation services	Better than basic primary care services	A few major programmes	Good or excellent leadership	Higher budget allocation relative to target	Lower internal migration
GAP NARROWING	1	1	1	0	1	0	1
	2	1	1	1	1	1	0
	3	1	1	0	1	1	0
	4	1	1	0	1	1	0
	5	1	1	1	1	1	0
	6	1	1	1	0	1	1
	7	1	1	0	1	1	1
	8	0	1	1	1	1	0
	9	1	0	0	1	0	1
	10	1	0	0	1	0	1
	11	1	0	0	1	0	1
	12	No data	1	1	0	1	0
	13	0	0	No data	0	1	0
GAP NOT NARROWING	14	1	1	0	1	1	1
	15	0	1	1	0	1	0
	16	0	1	0	1	0	0
	17	1	0	0	1	0	0
	18	1	0	0	1	0	0
	19	1	0	0	1	0	0
	20	1	0	0	0	0	0
	21	0	0	0	0	0	0
	22	No data	0	0	1	0	0
	23	1	0	0	1	1	1
	24	1	0	0	1	1	0
	25	1	0	0	1	0	1
	26	0	0	0	0	1	0
	27	1	0	0	0	1	0

Key:

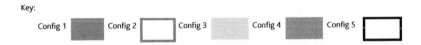

Config 1　　Config 2　　Config 3　　Config 4　　Config 5

identified. However, good/exemplary primary care services appear to be very important for positive outcomes in this field: they feature in nine of the 13 cases with a narrowing outcome. All three narrowing combinations shown in Table 8.2 are quite close to being sufficient, with few contradictory cases. The first combination combines a PCT budget allocation closer to target with good/exemplary primary care services. It includes eight narrowing cases and two contradictory not narrowing cases. The higher budget condition applied when a case was receiving no less than 4.3% under their target budget as assessed by the DH, using a needs–based formula. Although PCTs below target were being lifted towards it over time, many still faced a backlog of under-resourcing during the period covered by our study (House of Commons Health Committee, 2009). The second combination combines good or exemplary smoking cessation services with good or exemplary primary care services, with seven narrowing cases and one contradictory case. Good or exemplary smoking cessation services also appear in the third, more complex, combination, although this only has three narrowing cases together with one contradictory case.

The two combinations with an outcome of not narrowing the CVD gap both include 'no major programmes'. This cannot be judged a necessary condition because it appears in one of the narrowing combinations, but combined with a PCT budget that is further from target and higher population turnover as indicated by the population migration condition, it is sufficient for the outcome to be not narrowing, with seven cases and no contradictions. The second not narrowing combination, combining no major programmes with basic primary care services, includes 11 cases without a narrowing gap but three contradictory narrowing cases.

Teenage conceptions[57]

There are two narrowing configurations in Table 8.3. More detailed descriptions of these conditions are found in Appendix B. In the first configuration there is just one sufficient condition for the narrowing outcome to be present: when the case has a higher minority ethnic population as a proportion of the total population. This is not, however, a necessary condition because it is not present in the second narrowing configuration. Instead, this comprises a combination of lower numbers in drug treatment, a higher proportion of under-18s and a 'basic' standard of commissioning. This is sufficient for a narrowing gap to be present, without the apparent advantage of a higher proportion of minority ethnic groups, but none of the conditions on their own are necessary: what matters is the combination, and this is sufficient for a narrowing gap. As with the cancers results, a basic rather than a good or exemplary standard of commissioning is a surprising and counter-intuitive relationship with the narrowing of health inequality gaps.

Turning to the not narrowing configurations, three combinations of conditions were identified as being sufficient for the not narrowing outcome in the case of teenage conceptions. The first is a combination of a lower proportion of minority ethnic groups in the population and a lower proportion of under-18s. The second is a combination of a lower proportion of minority ethnic groups in the population

Table 8.3: Conditions associated with a narrowing gap for teenage conceptions (1= present; 0= absent)

	Area	Higher BMEs	Lower drug treatment	Higher under 18s	Basic commissioning of services	Fair, poor or mixed leadership	Intervention focuses on community settings	Major programmes	Lower deprivation	Higher educational achievement
GAP NARROWING	1	1	1	1	1	1	1	1	1	1
	2	1	0	1	0	0	0	0	0	0
	3	1	0	1	0	0	1	1	1	1
	4	1	0	1	1	1	0	0	0	0
	5	1	1	0	1	1	1	0	0	0
	6	1	1	0	1	1	0	0	0	0
	7	1	1	0	1	1	0	1	0	1
	8	1	1	0	0	1	1	1	0	0
	9	0	1	1	1	1	1	1	1	0
	10	0	1	1	1	1	1	1	0	0
	11	0	1	1	1	1	0	0	1	1
GAP NOT NARROWING	12	0	1	0	0	0	0	0	1	0
	13	0	1	0	1	1	1	0	1	1
	14	0	1	0	0	0	0	0	1	1
	15	0	1	0	1	0	0	1	1	1
	16	0	1	0	0	0	0	0	0	1
	17	0	1	0	0	0	0	0	0	0
	18	0	0	0	1	1	1	0	1	1
	19	0	0	0	1	0	0	0	1	1
	20	0	0	0	0	0	1	0	1	1
	21	0	0	1	1	1	1	0	1	1
	22	0	0	1	1	1	0	0	0	0
	23	0	0	0	1	0	0	0	0	1
	24	0	0	0	0	0	1	1	0	0
	25	0	0	0	1	1	0	0	0	0
	26	0	1	1	0	0	1	0	0	0
	27	0	1	0	0	1	0	1	1	0

Key:
Config 1 ☐   Config 2 ▨   Config 3 ▨   Config 4 ▨   Config 5 ☐

and higher numbers in drug treatment. The third is a combination of a lower proportion of minority ethnic groups in the population and a good or exemplary standard of commissioning. It is not surprising to see the presence of a lower proportion of minority ethnic groups in the population associated with a not narrowing gap, given the makeup of the two narrowing sets above. This condition is necessary for the outcome of not narrowing to be present in any of the three configurations, but it is not sufficient on its own.

Discussion

QCA is a useful type of analysis for policy makers and practitioners because it points to conditions and important combinations of conditions in ways that can be acted upon. QCA offers a possible strategy for isolating the key drivers of change in their combinations, capturing the importance of both interventions and context case by case, rather than estimating the effects of individual variables averaged across all cases. Our study was partly intended to be a tool (a tin-opener) for practitioners to use to consider patterns in ways of working and local contextual conditions. The results from this study can be regarded as providing both a basis for further investigation and indications for the direction of future action. For instance, taking the example of the CVD inequality gap, good smoking cessation services, good primary care services, good leadership and a PCT budget allocation close to target were identified as associated with this gap narrowing over a time horizon of a few years. This can be used either by areas without these attributes as justification for prioritising improvement and investment in these factors, or as a basis for learning from areas that have assessed their situation as better in these respects. It is important to note, however, that our findings, albeit based on substantive and theoretical reasoning, must be regarded as associations between conditions and outcomes rather than clear demonstrations of causation. Consequently, follow-up evaluation needs to be part of any such learning process. By looking at how conditions combined, the study also points to the importance of local contexts for tackling health inequalities. The PCT being close or at its target budget allocation was an important contextual condition for narrowing the cancer and CVD gaps. Higher internal migration was associated with not narrowing the CVD gap.

The counter-intuitive findings were initially puzzling, but the way that the conditions involved all related to bureaucratic work suggested an explanation connected with distracting from operational work on the ground. It was interesting in this respect that for cancers we found that there was an inverse relationship between individual commitment and championing on the one hand and these 'bureaucratic' conditions on the other. This is not to suggest that practices such as partnership working, workforce planning and monitoring are not important, but that too much focus on these activities may be counter-productive. It was fascinating to find from our practitioner workshops that this explanation often chimed with local experience, and examples were recounted of how overweening management and planning processes distracted from what practitioners felt really mattered. It is echoed in

Travers' (2007) study of 'the new bureaucracy'. Audit culture is a prime example of this, including taking time from 'normal work' without adding anything (Clarke, 2006). Appendix C shows the descriptors used to assess our 'bureaucratic conditions'. They were drafted on the assumption that good is better than basic, and so on. Looking at these descriptors through the lens of the above discussion, we might indeed interpret 'basic' as having the tools for the job in place, while the good and exemplary descriptors have a strong emphasis on plans, strategies, contracts, targets and progress reviews. Our results suggest that not only does this bureaucratic work not matter, it actually worsens outcomes. Seddon (2005; 2008) has explored this issue, arguing that audit culture focuses systems on compliance with targets and prescribed processes rather than learning how to match capability to outcomes. Achieving good or exemplary performance with processes of commissioning, workforce planning, strategic partnership working and reviewing is likely to entail an opportunity cost of time and resources that could otherwise be focused on 'normal work'. That normal work in the second set combination of the teenage conceptions results appears to have something to do with effective diversion from risky behaviours, in areas where under-18s make up a higher proportion of the local population and services may therefore have the critical mass needed for this kind of impact.

The way that some of our results questioned received wisdom such as devoting substantial resources to partnership working or focusing teenage pregnancy interventions in school rather than community settings was often validated by practitioners' experiential knowledge, although not without dissent. The benefit of QCA was to recognise the complexity of these practitioners' experiences, while also establishing a focus on clearly defined conditions and their relationships with outcomes. Too often either complexity is recognised in narrative 'good practice' case studies but without systematic comparison of these practices in combination with other factors, or systematic comparison is undertaken using quantitative techniques that generalise from relationships between variables rather than the conditions that apply in real world cases.

It is interesting that the cancer and CVD configurations in particular are so different. For cancer, tackling inequalities is recognised as needing 'clear commitment across the patient pathway at every level of NHS [National Health Service] cancer services' (National Cancer Inequality Initiative, 2010: 27). The National Cancer Plan, published in 2000, inherited a situation where 'patients often waited unacceptably long periods for diagnosis and treatment, coordination of care between all the health care professionals involved in cancer was often lacking and standards of care varied widely across the country' (Richards, 2007: 1). The plan represented a determination to improve cancer services and invest in ending inequalities of access to cancer care resulting from a failure to detect and treat early and quickly (DH, 2000b). While deprivation and lifestyle factors are acknowledged, the emphasis on earlier detection by expanding screening and awareness programmes, and on timely and more effective treatment, is very strong. This creates a context that would legitimise the arguments of determined clinical champions for focusing the increased flow of resources into reshaping services, finding cancers in areas of high prevalence and channelling cases into treatment. The substantial increase in the number of cancers diagnosed and rising survival rates means that these medical interventions must be credited with saving many potential premature deaths (Richards, 2007). Bureaucratic practices taken beyond what is necessary appear to hinder this, whether by diverting time and effort or by inhibiting championing itself. A recent review notes the progress made with tackling cancer but also draws attention to the continuing inequalities in cancer outcomes (National Cancer Inequality Initiative, 2010). Our analysis suggests some possible reasons for their persistence.

Tackling cancer inequalities across the whole care pathway was an established agenda at the time of our data collection, championed by a National Cancer Director and, we suggest, also depending on local championing across local health systems. There was no equivalent call to reshape services across the pathway for CVD. The national service framework for coronary heart disease, published in 2000, required primary care organisations to establish preventive services based on identifying and treating people with established disease or risk factors (DH, 2000a). Given free primary care coverage in England and the availability of drugs such as statins and anti-hypertensives that can successfully manage CVD risk factors, as well as the availability of free smoking cessation services either directly or through referral, this comprehensive approach to detection and treatment in primary care was a sensible strategy. However, the response from primary care – run in the UK largely by self-employed general practitioners (GPs) – was variable. Subsequent research identified the importance of the quality of primary care services across an area in achieving a reduction in CVD inequalities. It called on PCTs to ensure that the quality and quantity of primary care in deprived areas meets need and is well-organised, including challenging GP practices causing concern (Ali et al, 2008; Bentley, 2008; Care Quality Commission, 2009).

It is, therefore, not surprising that we see good or exemplary primary care services in two of the three configurations with a narrowing outcome for CVD. The good or exemplary smoking cessation services condition is also present in two configurations. While these services might be thought to associate with the cancer outcome as well, the effect of smoking cessation on cancer mortality is likely to be more long term than for CVD, and smoking cessation services have been authoritatively identified as critically important to achieving a reduction in CVD mortality in deprived areas (Marmot, 2010). However, as with primary care services, there is geographical variation in the effectiveness of services (NAO, 2010).

For the teenage conceptions study the result for the proportion of minority ethnic groups in the population condition is striking. In the narrowing set, this is a single sufficient condition. The presence of a higher proportion of minority ethnic groups in the population to start with appears to be associated with the narrowing gap. This conclusion is supported by the presence of lower minority ethnic group representation in the populations of all the areas with not narrowing outcomes. Consequently, lower proportions of minority ethnic groups in the population can be considered a *necessary* condition for not narrowing outcomes among the participating group of Spearhead areas. This finding is discussed further below, in relation to implications for policy and practice.

Implications for policy and practice

Cancers

It appears that among the group of Spearhead area participants in the study, action to tackle cancer mortality inequalities needed the individual commitment of cancer champions. Although this was not sufficient on its own, among our group of Spearhead PCTs it was necessary in all the configurations with a narrowing cancer gap and absent in all the configurations where the cancer gap is not narrowing. Stocking's (1985) study of innovation in the NHS found that champions often had a key role in getting new approaches to problems taken up and, crucially, diffused across the system. Many subsequent studies have identified the role of champions in developing and disseminating process improvements and best practices across networks, including preventive care (Ballard et al, 2007), integrated service delivery (Kathol et al, 2010) and pharmacy-based interventions (Westrick and Breland, 2009). Zöllner (2002) and Marmot (2010) both argue for championing as necessary for progress in reducing health inequalities. In discussions with practitioners at the workshops about the questionnaire design and discussion of the results, championing of early detection and treatment was said to be key. This factor was seen to be linked with the role of cancer networks. The NHS Cancer Plan put local cancer networks at the heart of a commitment to tackle cancer and called for them to be strongly led and to target resources where most needed (DH, 2000b). Local champions are likely to have a crucial influence, concentrating spending on higher rates of early detection and treatment, with this likely to be effective in reducing premature mortality.

Our findings also suggest that spending on tackling these inequalities should be high enough. We found the key threshold to be at least £86 per head, based on net expenditure in 2005/06. This level of spending is not enough on its own, however: rather, it needs to be associated with effective championing. Nonetheless, the nature and direction of that relationship remains unclear from our findings, since we cannot say whether higher spending is because of championing or whether higher spending is a precondition for successful championing, only that the two go together. Championing combined with higher spending on cancer programmes (above our binarisation threshold) appeared to be a very focused and effective combination.

It further appears that localities should avoid developing processes to excess, such as the bureaucracy of partnership meetings, writing (rather than delivering) plans and frequent monitoring. Process is not unimportant, but too much focus on plans and strategies may detract from focusing on actions that have a direct impact on the cancer gap. The first evidence for the potentially negative effect of bureaucracy was in the narrowing configurations where the public health workforce and monitoring were basic rather than the good or exemplary assessments that might be expected. In one of the not narrowing configurations we saw what we suggest are two similar bureaucratic conditions combining with a good or exemplary public health workforce: good or exemplary commissioning and good or exemplary strategic partnership working. We suggest that these attributes are 'bureaucratic conditions' because they can entail considerable effort devoted to meetings, plans and paperwork. This leads us to a recommendation that intensive work of this kind should be avoided, as it may distract effort from a focus on the cancer gap. It is important here to note that the 'basic' descriptors for commissioning, partnership working and the public health workforce were not undemanding, and no area assessed these as less than basic. The idea that being 'better' than basic could be dysfunctional found support among many of the practitioners in our workshops.

Wider determinants of inequalities in cancer mortality also appeared to be important and to make a difference locally. Local partners should work together to tackle high deprivation and crime rates, in particular. We found thresholds at a 2007 Index of Multiple Deprivation score of 31.5 or higher and a crime rate of 64.5 offences per 1,000 population or higher, suggesting it is – in relative terms – very high deprivation and crime rates that presented the most important challenges in terms of contextual or environmental conditions for some Spearhead areas.

National policy was not the focus of our study but some issues should be noted. The role of local cancer inequality champions could be formalised and supported. Clinical commissioning groups (CCGs), as successors to PCTs, that have large gaps in cancers inequalities could be encouraged, and supported, to increase their spending per head on cancer. Our evidence also suggests that there should be a sharper focus in national policy on enabling localities to reduce very high deprivation and very high crime rates. Finally, given the strength of the counter-intuitive findings in this report, national government should ensure that performance management does not encourage excessive process management locally.

CVD

Our results suggest a number of improvements in management and practice that local agencies could seek to make as a contribution to closing the gaps between areas in outcomes for CVD. First, smoking cessation services should operate at least to the standard for good service specified in our descriptor: that is, provision is mapped across the area and is available in a wide range of settings; prevalence data is collected and used to target services; and there is effective targeting of 'seldom seen, seldom heard' groups. Particular attention should be paid to good leadership of this work. Appendix B gives more details of the descriptors involved. Second, primary care services should be at least up to the standard in our descriptor for good services: active management of Quality and Outcomes Framework (QOF) exception reporting by CCGs; primary care working with other services to reach vulnerable groups and actively seek out people with (or at risk of) disease; and the quantity of primary care in local areas meeting local needs. Particular attention should be paid to good leadership of this work. Again, Appendix B also gives more details of the descriptors involved. Third, areas with higher levels of population churn (we found 3.6% inflow and 4% outflow to be important thresholds) and total PCT budget allocations still below target (we found more than 4.3%

below target to be an important threshold) should be aware that these may be significant barriers to narrowing their CVD gaps. Measures to improve population stability or more effectively reach mobile sections of the population should be considered; and performance–management processes should recognise the possible relationship between distance from target and the extent to which relevant health inequalities outcomes can be attained.

National policy implications arising from this study include targeting support to bring smoking cessation and primary care services up to the standard of the 'good' and preferably 'exemplary' descriptor, and supporting leadership development to make this happen locally. Our evidence also suggested that all Spearhead areas needed their PCT budgets to be at or very close to their target budget allocations. During the research we argued that this might have been especially important for areas with relatively high population mobility. This finding may be significant under the new health and social care arrangements, following concerns (see Turner et al, 2013, for example) about the potential lack of engagement among clinical commissioners with population health, compared with patient, perspectives. If these concerns are borne out there is an even greater role for health and wellbeing boards (HWBs) and joint strategic needs assessments (JSNAs) to ensure that areas with higher levels of population mobility take an integrated approach to understanding local population dynamics in planning and delivering services.

Teenage conceptions

There is evidence that teenage conception rates have been relatively high among young people from some minority ethnic backgrounds (French et al, 2005; Teenage Pregnancy Unit, 2005). While no evidence could be identified from the research or policy literature of faster progress with reducing rates among these groups, our results suggest that this may be what has been happening. We can only speculate about the reasons: increased awareness of the risk of sexually transmitted infections and rising educational aspirations and achievements are possibilities. What is strange is that the issue has not received more attention. We note, for example, that the last government's review of England's national teenage pregnancy strategy has no consideration of ethnic factors (DCSF/DH, 2010).

Other interesting conditions that appear to be causal are the proportion of the local population in drug treatment and the proportion of under–18s. The former could be regarded as more than just an indicator of the level of substance misuse and to be tracing risk-taking generally, including teenage sexual behaviour, given that risky behaviours are known to cluster across domains (Seamark and Gray, 1998; Coleman, 2002). The under-18s condition is more difficult to interpret. A higher proportion of under-18s in the local population is associated with a narrowing gap and may mean that these areas are more likely to provide services for this group that divert young people from risk-taking, including local sexual health provision. Unfortunately, a services indicator of this type is not available, so this explanation has to remain speculative. What we can say is that there is something about a higher proportion of under-18s that appears to be associated with a narrowing of the teenage pregnancies gap, although only in combination with lower numbers in drug treatment and a basic standard of commissioning.

National policy implications flowing from these findings include encouraging a sharper focus on supporting those localities with lower proportions of minority ethnic groups, lower numbers of under-18s and higher numbers of those with substance misuse issues.

Overall learning and common threads

QCA is an exploratory method, based on logical arguments that are made explicit in relation to real cases and their complexity. Our analysis has identified complex associations between configurations of conditions on the one hand, and the narrowing or otherwise of inequalities in outcomes for cancers, CVD and teenage conceptions on the other. Within these complex patterns, we have inferred causal relationships from finding that conditions found in one configuration were absent or acted differently in other configurations. An important aspect of our findings was that different paths (combinations of conditions) could lead to the same outcome – or that the same outcome can be reached in different ways. The different paths in the results relate, in particular, to the cases that participated in the study. The research team provided a general report to all the participating areas, together with a section individual to each area identifying them in the results and providing a summary. This was intended to be a tin-opener to assist local policy makers and practitioners in the interpretation of progress towards narrowing health inequalities gaps. In addition, workshops with practitioners were held to interpret the findings, while facilitating learning exchanges between areas. In recognising these different paths as sets of the same type of cases, practitioners can (and did) make use of the results to consider strategies that best make sense for their area (Fiss, 2007).

Ragin (2000) asserts that necessary conditions have significant policy implications. Necessary conditions may both constrain and enable outcomes, but it is much more difficult to enable an outcome because all the necessary conditions must be in place. It only takes one of these to be absent for the outcome's achievement to be frustrated. It is perhaps surprising that in our analysis we identify a relatively small number of necessary conditions and configurations. Although these conditions are themselves quite complex, none is sufficient on its own, and there are alternative pathways to the same outcome, which adds further complexity. However, the state of many conditions often did not appear to matter to the outcome. In some cases, this may be because what matters is that a level of achievement for a practice is at least basic, and instances of Spearhead areas assessing any practices as that poor were very rare. So our analysis reflects practices being on the whole at least basic; it then picks out practices and other conditions where their qualitatively different states matter to the outcome. QCA, to quote Ragin (2000: 260) again, is 'a tool of discovery' rather than a hypothesis-testing technique. The causal arguments are based on association, but supported by substantive and theoretical arguments about necessity and sufficiency that apply to real cases and connect with actual practice. Indeed, returning to individual cases is an important dimension of QCA studies, either to understand anomalies or to develop general explanations. For example, although it was not possible within the scope of this study to explore further the services and risk diversion aspect that we suggest was traced by the drug treatment and under-18 conditions in the teenage conceptions analysis, the study creates a framework for doing this (and local policy makers and practitioners were encouraged to do so using the feedback provided with the final reports). We would expect to find better services for young people in the areas with lower numbers in drug treatment and higher under-18s in the local population, as well as commissioning that is 'good enough' but not so good that it distracts from delivering these services.

The study outlined here pioneered the use of QCA in exploring the key public health issue of health inequalities and how they can be narrowed. The results and recommendations should be read with suitable caution. Given the extent to which we rely on self-assessment in a relatively small group of localities, corroboration from other research will be important. This is particularly the case with regard to our intriguing counter-intuitive results and our theory that too much partnership working, planning and monitoring may be counter–productive for the dedicated and focused work needed to tackle health inequalities at a local level.

Conclusion

The evidence about health inequalities is relatively clear at an aggregate level. The significance of structural factors and the persistence of a social gradient in health are commonly cited (see, for example, Black, 1980; Graham and Kelly, 2004; Sassi, 2005; Marmot, 2010; Wilkinson and Pickett, 2010; Dorling, 2013b) as significant factors in continuing health inequalities in England. It is also clear from our results and other studies (see, for example, Bambra, 2012; Vizard and Obolenskaya, 2013) that progress can be achieved by some areas for certain aspects of health inequalities, notably infant mortality and life expectancy for cancers and circulatory diseases, particularly when measured in terms of absolute rather than relative gaps. What this chapter shows is how policy and practice interact with context among a group of deprived English local authority areas in terms of the variations in progress towards health inequalities targets. This study does not offer a complete understanding of progress towards narrowing health inequalities gaps, but shows how a variety of conditions interact over a (relatively short) period of time across these areas. This enabled the research team to develop set-theoretic knowledge about these cases and use this as a tin–opener to explore what may be associated with improvement or non–improvement towards narrowing health inequality gaps.

Rihoux and Lobe (2009) describe the QCA process as a 'funnel of complexity', through which a key enterprise is to reduce the inherent complexity of cases to some level of parsimony. In the study described above we were able to use QCA to develop set-theoretic knowledge but not to the extent of the fullest iterations of QCA: truth tables and a Boolean minimisation. A truth table would produce a table of cases grouped into configurations, as opposed to the dichotomised data tables (see Tables 8.1–8.3) that formed the basis of our results, and a Boolean minimisation would reduce these further to a number of parsimonious equations or formulas derived from the conditions in the configurations (see Rihoux and Lobe, 2009; Rihoux and De Meur, 2009, for further details). Our apparently more simplistic and less advanced (in terms of the formal stages of a QCA exercise) results might, therefore, appear to be a limitation of the study, and certainly would if they were not properly qualified. However, one interpretation of the research is that the results can be viewed as demonstrating the complexity of health inequalities in local systems. QCA is regarded as a method that is oriented towards complexity (see Buijs et al, 2009, for example). While the method does not answer the question set[58] with as much certainty or as neatly as we might have liked by providing more parsimonious configurations and equations, it does allow us to see the complexity of the issue at hand through the combinations of conditions identified here. It also provides the tools and framework for researchers, policy makers and practitioners to interpret these results alongside more detailed local knowledge about the functioning of these local systems. This is what Rihoux and Lobe (2009) describe as the 'downstream: interpretation' phase of QCA and forms the latter stages of the funnel of complexity. By acknowledging and accepting the complexity of health inequalities, and that we are not going to reduce the social world into neatly defined boxes, applied research such as this can help to add further certainty to our understanding by, somewhat paradoxically, accepting that our knowledge is often imperfect and uncertain, and requires collaboration between different types of knowledge, as suggested by Head (2007).

NINE

Conclusions

Introduction

> Ill-health is a manifestation of disordered biology but
> these biological processes are influenced by the conditions
> in which people are born, grow, live, work and age, and
> inequalities in power, money and resources that give
> rise to inequities in conditions of daily life – the social
> determinants of health. Just as biological sciences are
> important to understanding health, so are the social sciences.
> (Marmot, 2014: 6)

We agree, and hope that this book has gone some way towards
contributing to how social sciences can enhance our understandings
of health and health inequalities. This concluding chapter will draw
the discussion to a close by discussing three key issues that have arisen
over the course of the book: the role of the National Health Service
(NHS) and others in tackling health inequalities; governance of health
inequalities; and methodological and ideological considerations. Before
we begin this discussion it is useful to briefly recap on the extent of
health inequalities in England, drawing on the latest available data at
the time of writing.

Vizard and Obolenskaya (2013) state that deep inequalities remain
in health outcomes in England, despite some improvements in health
outcomes when measured in terms of absolute rather than relative
gaps.[59] They continue to contend that, with one year's data still
outstanding, the New Labour targets to reduce the absolute gap in
mortality inequality for circulatory disease and cancers are on course
to be met, and so is the target for the reduction in infant mortality.
However, the target to reduce life expectancy inequalities for men and
women in terms of reducing the relative gap between Spearhead areas
and the England average is not expected to be met, as both absolute
and relative gaps have increased. This latter target is most significant
to the health of the population overall, and we see that, despite
improvements in child, cancer and circulatory disease mortality rates,
people from Spearhead areas are on average living eight years less than

those in the least deprived fifth of areas (Vizard and Obolenskaya, 2013: 96). The same source also demonstrates that not only do people from poorer areas live shorter lives, a smaller proportion of their life is spent disability-free (74% compared with 85%: for Spearhead areas and the least deprived fifth of areas, respectively). As we argued earlier in the book (see Chapter Three, section on area-based approaches to tackling health inequalities, and Chapter Four, section on measurement and complexity, for example) life expectancy as a whole rather than falling mortality rates from a particular disease is a more complex matter, and relates to a combination of conditions that may be mutually intercausal and limiting to life.

The role of the NHS and others in tackling health inequalities

A strong theme running throughout the book has been the different ways that health and health inequalities can be conceptualised. In Chapter Five, Gerald Wistow asserted that the NHS was principally designed to provide universal personal medical services and can be seen as a diversion from providing health for all as opposed to health (medical) care for all. This we describe as a category error: it is one in which the dominant logic model is too narrowly focused to tackle the social and economic determinants of health inequalities. Indeed the National Audit Office (NAO) reports that the Department of Health (DH) itself has estimated that only around 15–20% of inequalities in mortality rates can be directly influenced by health interventions which prevent or reduce the risk of ill health (NAO, 2010). This appears to support our earlier argument that the NHS was primarily established as a sickness service, with resources and attention focused too much on responding to symptoms and too little on addressing underlying causes. This is essentially a tame solution to a wicked problem, and one that is closely associated with the medical model. This is not to argue that medicine and the medical model has no role – far from it – but that it should be restricted if health inequalities are a high priority.

It is encouraging that the President of the UK Faculty of Public Health, Professor John Ashton, was quoted as identifying the biggest public health challenge as being:

> growing inequalities in people's position, income and control over their lives over the last 20 or 30 years. Lots of people are being left behind. Outside the wealthy parts of the country people are living miserable, short lives, with

a lot more ill-health than people in the more advantaged
parts of the country. (Campbell, 2014)

However, as we have already identified, there will be a rough 95%
to 5% split between NHS resource allocations and those for public
health in 2013/14. So while it is encouraging that health inequalities
remain a public health priority, public health must seek to influence
the NHS proportion of resource allocation. In so doing, the medical
model's concern to treat symptoms more than causes of ill health
needs to be challenged, and attention must be paid to the interplay
between individual agency and the underlying structural determinants
of health. Changing the logic model of the 95% (the NHS) of health
resource allocations is critical to tackling health inequalities. In this
respect, we can look back to the initial response of the government
and how the Public Health Act 1848 focused on the health of the
population, conceiving initiatives and interventions to improve the
public's health, which pre-dated the creation of the NHS and the long
shift to an offer of universal personal medical services by 100 years.
Changing the operating model of the NHS has proven to be largely
intractable, with the focus essentially on responding to symptoms rather
than causes of ill health. For example, Turner et al (2013: 6) found
that, despite some progress, practitioners recognised that primary care
trust (PCT) commissioning had failed to deliver significant progress
around reduced health inequalities. A key issue identified here was
the poor track record of PCTs in shifting resources out of secondary
care and into primary care and public health interventions that may
have an impact on health inequalities. Most commissioning work has
been concerned with the 'transactional' role of maintaining existing
contracts rather than a 'transformational' shift to other areas (Turner
et al, 2013: 6). Responsibility for the health inequalities agenda was
seen as primarily a responsibility for those with public health roles,
rather than a core commissioning responsibility.

Indeed, despite the Coalition accepting most of the Marmot
Review's recommendations, the rejection of the Review's prescription
to narrow income inequalities reinforces the lack of concern with
social and economic causes. This is consistent with official responses
to health inequalities continuing to fall short of the diagnosis of the
problem. Indeed, Davis et al identify a continued tension in local policy
between an 'essentially medicalized and minimal definition of care
and one in which care reaches beyond a group of people with critical
needs' (2011: 691). This, in turn, contributes to the organisation and
distribution of health systems, which is the focus of the next section.

The governance of health inequalities

The notion that health inequalities are a wicked problem has implications for the kinds of approaches that solve these. Grint states that we need 'to assume that no–one has the solution in isolation and that the problem is a system not an individual problem and not a problem caused by or solved by a single aspect of the system' (2008: 17). This complements Kooiman's general assertion about governance, that 'there has been great progress in the knowledge of parts, but much less in the knowledge of the relation between them, and the relation between parts and wholes' (2003: 197). Kooiman points out that governance is a mix of all kinds of governing efforts by all manner of social-political actors; and that different governance modes and orders are 'societal "responses" to persistent and changing governing "demands", set against ever growing societal diversity, dynamics and complexity' (2003: 3). Narrowing the concept down somewhat, Stoker defines governance as the 'complex set of institutions and actors that are drawn from but also beyond government' (1998: 19). Consequently, the concept of governance embraces a greater awareness of the need for the state to interact with other societal actors. In Chapter Two we identified service users as carers (both formal and informal); public, private, and voluntary service providers; advocacy groups; and commissioners and managers of services – these are different types of societal actors with a role in health inequalities. They operate and interact across a range of scales from local government to the neighbourhood level. This, in turn, implies the need to coordinate action across not only different sectors and scales but also multiple forms of knowledge including scientific, political and practical, which Head (2007) identifies as being essential for effective planning. As a consequence of these types of development, Kelly (2010) argues that public health needs to understand the linkages and interactions between different phenomena, and this requires both individual and social levels of explanation.

As we have already seen, the Black Report (1980) called for greater coordination between government departments in the administration of health-related policies at both national and local levels. This call for greater coordination was a recurring theme in the Acheson Report and Marmot Review, as well. These extended the need for coordination across different sectors, partly in response to the introduction of quasi-markets into the English public sector and partly through the growing rhetoric around the importance of community engagement and empowerment. The Marmot Review states that 'action is required across all these social determinants of health and needs to involve all central and local government departments as well as the third and private sectors. Action taken by the Department of Health and the NHS alone will not reduce health inequalities' (2010: 19). This reflects some of the complexity of solving health inequalities as a social problem, as it sits between different parts of government as well as with non-governmental actors. A further complicating factor identified by Grint (2008) is that, because it is a wicked problem, we do not know precisely what to do (if we did it would be a tame problem). As a result, coordination is made more difficult and may contribute to Turner et al's (2013) finding that policy statements and process documents reflecting an apparent commitment to addressing inequalities were often viewed as having little influence on action and tokenistic. Thus, without clearly defined responsibilities the intractability of health inequalities may be deterring action among stakeholders.

Grint, in his generally excellent critique of wicked problems, asserts that 'we need not worry about the role that 'Fatalists' might play in resolving Wicked Problems because by and large they don't [play a role]' (2008: 17). For Grint, the Fatalists are those that are lacking a group dimension and are isolated individuals who believe themselves to be undermined by the power of rules and roles. In terms of health inequalities, we might equate these with marginalised individuals who lack a 'stake' in society and exhibit unhealthy behaviours and lifestyles as a result. In other words, precisely the types of individuals that need to be part of the complex solution/s to the wicked problem of health inequalities. However, as we have already noted, it is not straightforward to develop these solutions. In fact, Green (as summarised in Warr et al, 2013: 97) identifies three trends in public health promotion that are reinforcing boundaries between public health professionals and disadvantaged place-based communities:

- A growing reliance on evidence-based policy and practice … is deeply embedded in professional knowledge and values that limits the active role that communities can play in developing and managing initiatives.
- The emphasis on inter-professional teams, multi-agency partnerships and increasingly sophisticated knowledge construction (such as meta-analysis and systematic reviews) combine to ensure that public health practice and knowledge is consolidated as the preserve of professionals and inaccessible to lay communities.
- Professional expertise and competence are wielded to 'repair' perceived problems and deficits in communities,

which reaffirm the differences between professionals and communities.

In light of trends such as this, the HINST authors stated in Chapter Seven that even if the quality of services is good, if patients drop out and do not connect with them appropriately they will have little impact. In response, they provided the example of the 'Big Bolton Healthcheck' (see the section on practical illustrations), which was based in primary care but recruited support from across the local community, including health and social care frontline services, the voluntary sector and commercial pharmacies. As a result, a large proportion of previously unmet need was addressed through a governance solution to a wicked problem. A further example from Chapter Seven highlights an approach to tackling health inequalities that responds to what might be described as the potentially fatalist self-organising characteristics of members of local systems through focusing on the importance of supported self-care. The argument here is that if care packages are not used appropriately by patients then outcomes will be limited, however potentially effective the planned treatment was. Consequently, the interactions between service providers and patients need to be closely monitored and managed because there may be a wide variety of reasons why treatment plans are not being followed.

Alongside health and wellbeing boards (HWBs), joint strategic needs assessments (JSNAs) are important vehicles for coordinating action around health inequalities. The RSPH (2014) highlights that JSNAs are key to deciding the nature of the challenges to be addressed, deciding how best to respond, and who should implement the response. However, Turner et al (2013) identified concerns among practitioners about the impact of JSNAs in influencing mainstream commissioning action in relation to health inequalities, particularly because this is a joint responsibility, which may lead to a lack of ownership. One possible way forward, identified in Chapter Seven, was to view the JSNA as a process, not a document (or website). Findings should ideally move from dry analysis to 'marketing' the findings to a range of audiences (elected members; local authority officers; general practitioner (GP) commissioners; HealthWatch and the public). In so doing, JSNAs should consider the balance between the three categories of causes of health inequalities identified by the NAO (2010) – wider determinants, the lives people lead and the health services people use – in their local contexts. Indeed, trying to link inequalities to individual care pathways, where the emphasis is on keeping people out of care systems rather than facilitating entry and guiding them through (except where prevention fails), could be key to reframing health inequality challenges and deciding how to respond to these. This raises questions about how far you can go in the face of structurally embedded inequalities and the limits of public health-oriented care planning, but also exposes those influences at the level of individuals and draws attention to their personal narratives.

Methodological and ideological considerations

We begin this section by reflecting on the persistence of health inequalities and what is known about this. In this respect, Bambra et al contend that:

> in terms of the Marmot Review, it is on the one hand reassuring and on the other rather worrying that its recommendations continue to emphasise many of the same issues as the two previous reports [the Black and Acheson Reports]. For while it suggests that a relatively clear consensus about what needs to be done to tackle health inequalities has emerged, it also suggests, as others have claimed, that the impact of earlier research into health inequalities ... has actually had very little real impact on the types of policy implemented. (2011: 403)

This concluding section of the book will briefly consider two important themes that have recurred throughout and have important implications for both how we study health inequalities and why there may have been limited impact from the policies that have been implemented. The first theme is concerned with methodology and relates to how we understand health inequalities and the methods used to develop this understanding. These, in turn, have practical implications for addressing health inequalities because, as we have argued earlier, what has been done in practice to solve health inequalities relates to how these have been framed. The second theme focuses on how health inequalities relate to ideological considerations about the nature of society.

Our argument has been that the dominant strand in shaping policies to tackle health inequalities has been based on a category error, and that as a result the logic model adopted for understanding and addressing health inequalities has tended to mirror the medical model's concern to treat symptoms more than causes, giving too little attention to the interplay between individual agency and the underlying structural determinants of health. Here, Grint's discussion of wicked problems is very useful and draws our attention to the inordinate amount of time and money spent by the NHS on trying to change itself. He points out that very often that change has led to little more than restructuring or relabeling of the organisation rather than any radical attempt to rethink the purpose and realign it on that basis (2008: 11). It is useful to return to Rosen's (1987) distinction between simple and complex systems here. The former relates to a context in which a notion of state can be assigned once and for all and causal categories can be independently segregated from one another. The medical model's focus on measuring components as discrete elements, rather than elements of a dynamic and integrated system, is too closely aligned to Rosen's notion of simple systems to address the complexity of health inequalities, and the NHS needs radical realignment rather than organisational restructuring to do so.

A further methodological consideration identified by Curtis is that 'the context in which research has been carried out is often important. It is not necessarily appropriate to "project" information about how to reduce health inequalities drawn from research on certain groups of individuals in particular places to other populations in different settings' (2008: 300). For example, the seven neighbourhood deprivation cluster types identified in Chapter Seven show how deprivation in an ex-mining community is likely to be different from that of a neighbourhood largely comprised of ethnic minorities or an inner-city estate. These different contexts are likely to require different approaches to tackle the local manifestations of health inequalities. To this we must add Curtis' (2008) argument that not all elements of civil society are as easy to engage in debates about health, with marginal groups (those who tend to experience inequalities in health most sharply) being especially hard to engage. Nathanson and Hopper (2010) suggest that the Marmot Review targeted early years to such an extent because adults are more likely to be resistant to the intrusions of health visitors/ trainers/champions (the panoply of street-level workers envisioned by Marmot as leading the health charge at the local level) than children. These are some of the dynamics that make up complex systems and relate to the interactions between individual and social levels of explanation for health inequalities. In other words, we need to avoid the reductionism of isolating human agency and structures, and instead concentrate on the interactions between these. As Cohn et al note, 'complex health interventions will always be highly variable in both character and form due to the dynamic nature of their constituent parts and the inevitable adaptations that emerge from their implementation in local contexts' (2013: 42).

Turning now to ideological considerations, and Nathanson (2007) has claimed that public health action requires a combination of three ingredients: perceived peril to the nation or social order, state interest and capacity, and advocacy group pressure. Despite some commitments to health inequalities under the Coalition government, these three things are generally absent in the current political climate (as Nathanson and Hopper (2010) conclude). Grint (2008) asserts that the social construction of a problem legitimates a particular form of authority. Health inequalities are not being defined as enough of a 'threat' (in Grint's terms) to lead to sufficient authority to foster the collective action needed to address them as a wicked problem. A key question emerging here is: to what extent does this reflect the accepted social contract between government and governed? How far is there, at least implicit, popular support[60] for the current structure and stratification of society, including relatively high levels of health inequalities?

Inequality in England is a product of post-industrial capitalism and the possessive individualist ideology. In which case, some level of inequalities in healthy life expectancy is inevitable and, in this view, it is an acceptable consequence of economic policy and should be recognised as such. The alternative is to support redistributive policies, and the evidence (see, for example, Sassi, 2005 and Rowlingson, 2011) is that this would reduce health inequalities. However, Dorling argues that 'both Conservative and Labour government policy has been largely symbolic and has failed to tackle the disparities in income and wealth that drive rising health inequalities as measured across society. Instead, more potent and redistributive policies are needed to initiate change and greater equality' (2013a: 28). Nevertheless, Clarke and Newman (2012) suggest that equity and solidarity are being renegotiated through competing political discourses, and that a profound and deepening inequality of sacrifice between 'ordinary' people and a 'feral elite' is emerging. This is particularly troubling because, as Dorling (2013a: 7) notes, a key difference between the affluent now and in the 1930s is that the awareness of inequalities is much more prevalent in affluent groups; in the past, inequalities in premature mortality might have been viewed as an act of God, rather than a preventable tragedy.

Alongside the role of elites and the affluent there appears to be a collective apathy among the wider public about the need to redistribute wealth. For example, Clarke and Newman (2012) cite Rawnsley to point out that what matters in the minds of voters is which party will be viewed as the most competent in managing the economy, and that the restoration of 'business as usual' would, therefore, retain its dominance over any popular interventions to rein in the excesses of capitalism.

Indeed, Lupton et al found that 'two thirds of the population polled in the British election study favoured either the status quo in terms of tax and spend (56%), or cutting taxes and spending less (10%)' (2013: 8). Consequently, the social contract does not appear to be aligned with the Marmot Review's ambition to 'flatten the social gradient' (Nathanson and Hopper, 2010). Does this matter? Should we accept the 'general will' to maintain the status quo? Our argument is that yes, this does matter and we should not accept the status quo. Health is 'a state of complete physical, mental and social well-being' (WHO, 1948). Thus, inequalities in health are profoundly important to people's quality, and extent, of life and should form a key part of the social contract – that is, people's stake in society is intrinsically tied to their health. An equitable society is, therefore, one in which good health is evenly distributed across different social groups and does not follow a divisive social gradient.

If we want to see a more equitable society in terms of health outcomes then we need to respond to Burawoy's (2005) tension between policy sociology and critical sociology. Our argument is that we can do so, first, by changing how we conceptualise health inequalities as a policy problem; and second, by challenging the fundamental characteristics of society and the socially structured nature of health. In terms of the former, we have noted that understanding health inequalities and the determinants of these as intersecting complex systems at different levels can help identify ways in which interventions can make a difference. In so doing, a better understanding of exposure to risks leading to health inequalities can be developed and lead to perspectives that can inform and help structure a shift to intervening as far upstream as possible. The latter requires a change in the dominant organising principles of society to move towards more collectivist social norms and away from neoliberal economics and policies. Given the current scope of political debate in England, there seems limited potential to move away from a neoliberal economic model. Rather, the debate is around the how much social support and social investment will be grafted onto this, which matters in the extent to which equality is promoted or not within this model. This is, nonetheless, a disappointingly narrow ideological debate. However, it is probably wise to conclude our discussion on a positive note and we do so by returning to complexity and policy sociology. In Chapter Five we introduced the notion of equifinality, which is the idea that outcomes can be the product of multiple and different causal complexes, or that the same outcome can be reached in different ways, and this was illustrated in practice through the qualitative comparative analysis (QCA) study in Chapter Eight. Consequently, we can conclude that despite the overall significance of the structural determinants of health at an aggregate level, progress has been made in relation to some health inequality targets, and some localities with high levels of deprivation have made better progress in closing health inequalities gaps than others. This points us to the significance of local policies and the agency and reflexivity of social systems in tackling, or at least limiting, health inequalities.

Notes

1. The views expressed in this book are those of the authors and do not necessarily reflect the views of the NHS or Department of Health.
2. It is also important to note the emphasis placed at the end of the Labour period of government on preventative treatment such as statins and anti-hypertensives.
3. Ron Swanson is a fictional character in Parks and Recreation. He is the Director of the Parks and Recreation Department in Pawnee. As a libertarian he believes in a very small government and that the state should have a minimal role in telling people what to do or how we should lead our lives.
4. Although it should also be noted that the agency of individuals is an important factor in the construction of social reality; this is something we return to later in this chapter.
5. Shaw and Dorling (2004) define need as the geographical distribution of people both suffering poor health and living with a limiting long-term illness.
6. Ron Swanson sits in an extreme (to European eyes) libertarian tradition of this.
7. Hutton is here referring to Britain in the pre-enlargement Europe, but it is important to recognise that there are some much more minimal welfare states than Britain worldwide.
8. A measure of inequality among the values of a frequency distribution (such as income), in which 0 equals perfect equality and 1 is maximal inequality.
9. This may be due to a lack of education, depression, lifestyle choices and so on
10. The argument here is not against these methods *per se*, but against a hierarchy that excludes non-experimental forms of evidence.
11. Or rather how this is distributed across a heterogeneous group of marginalised in society.
12. We use the QCA term 'conditions' rather than Lazarsfeld's 'attributes'.
13. The questionnaires are available at: www.dur.ac.uk/spearheads.health/questionnaires.htm
14. The Quality and Outcomes Framework is an annual reward and incentive programme detailing general practitioner (GP) achievement results for managing chronic diseases, practice organisation, patient experience and extra services.
15. Most of these indicators were sourced from DCLG at: www.communities.gov.uk/communities/neighbourhoodrenewal/deprivation/deprivation07/.
16. In complexity terms we describe this as changes in the possible attractor sets within a state space of possibilities.
17. The other comparator was always infant mortality rates.
18. Now that taxes are in practice only for the little people – that is, the 90%+ of us who cannot engage in systematic tax avoidance.
19. The author has constantly to explain to students that a life expectancy at birth in the mid-nineteenth century of 40 years did not mean that everybody died at 40.

There were lots of old people about. Of course, there remain differences in infant and child mortality. Globally there are profound differences between societies that have undergone the health transition and those that have not. However, in developed societies – although there is, for example, a clear class gradient in infant mortality – the absolute numbers are so small that it is worthwhile asking if this is a useful measure. Inverting the measure and looking at survival rates gives differences by class that are now small, compared with relatively recent history.

[20] Age-related matters. The author, who is a regular swimmer, appreciates that teenagers can generally swim faster than him but does not like being passed repeatedly by young women in bikinis (a one piece indicates a serious swimmer) who swim with their heads out of the water. Such is life.

[21] The author is British – we can disregard the notion that in his case 'peoples' refers to Gael and Cymru with a pure Gael father and a half Gael and half Cymru mother.

[22] These are, in part, concessions to the strict Marxist conception of classes in terms of control/ownership of the means of production.

[23] For example, during the operating life of the Norwood Coke Works, inhabitants of central Gateshead regularly suffered from 'the Gateshead throat' in winter when the combination of domestic coal smoke and the coke works' fumes caused very considerable air pollution. Smoke control and the demolition of the coke works have much improved air quality, but if you lived in central Gateshead before those changes then there is a potential residual impact of those historic local causal powers in terms of your health state.

[24] And, of course, households.

[25] A measure of inequality among the values of a frequency distribution (such as income), in which 0 equals perfect equality and 1 is maximal inequality.

[26] Even 20 years ago the author's older daughter, aged 21 with a 2.1 in Economics from a Russell group university, got much the same sort of clerical administrative job as her grandmother had obtained some 50 years earlier at 16 with a school certificate.

[27] Particularly patients who might sue health providers.

[28] The practice may be much more of an issue.

[29] Byrne (2002) expands on this issue in some detail.

[30] Although even here there was, of course, a complex association with smoking.

[31] Stencil copying.

[32] Although local examples of equitable resourcing through QOF can be found in Chapter Seven and in Figure 7.11, specifically.

[33] See Chapter Two (section on inequality).

[34] Robert Joyce of the IFS (Institute for Fiscal Studies) explains that this is due to wages dipping sharply and benefits being more stable and going to those on the lowest incomes (see Tom Clark in *The Guardian*, 2 July 2014)

[35] Difference in performance between the disadvantaged and reference groups.

[36] Performance in the disadvantaged group as a proportion of performance in the reference group.

[37] Absolute gaps can narrow while relative gaps widen. Here, Spearhead areas closed the *difference* between themselves and the national average, but the performance of Spearhead areas as a *proportion* of the performance in the national average widened.

[38] For a fuller account of the impact of this on social and economic systems see Byrne (2005).

[39] Apart from London, which increased by 0.3%.

[40] And, following the Health and Social Care Act 2012, the public health function, which is discussed in more detail in the later section of Chapter Six on implications of health inequalities.

[41] Under New Labour this included such initiatives as Neighbourhood Renewal, New Deal for Communities and Total Place.

[42] The programme is available to view on YouTube: https://www.youtube.com/watch?v=CXWJ4GfQ22E

[43] The body formed out of the Marmot Review team.

[44] Respondents were professionals involved with health and social care commissioning at national and local levels.

[45] This diagram and those following in this chapter have been published previously in a Department of Health resource pack of best practice guidance (DH, (2010) Redoubling efforts to achieve the 2010 National Health Inequalities Life Expectancy Target, Gateway reference 13785).

[46] Tom Hennell, Senior Public Health Analyst, Department of Health North West, Narrowing the health inequalities gap: What went right and what went wrong?, in Symposium: 'Where next for health inequalities research?', 5–6 December 2012.

[47] A comprehensive range of tools to facilitate improvement of pathway design and management is available on the NHS Institute for Innovation and Improvement website, available at: www.institute.nhs.uk/option,com_quality_and_service_improvement_tools/Itemid,5015.html.

[48] An example pdf of the Merseyside and Cheshire Cancer Network tools is available at: www.mccn.nhs.uk/index.php/groups/view/id/14

[49] For more information on the HINST approach to reducing health inequalities due to cancer, see the report produced through the collaboration with the National Cancer Action Team: *How to reduce excess mortality from cancer in areas with the worst health and highest levels of deprivation*, available at: http://ncat.nhs.uk/sites/default/files/work-docs/HINST%20NCAT%20How%20to%20Cancer%20final%20_%2009032011.pdf.

[50] As such, the findings presented here relate to a particular period in time but the application of the methodology to health inequalities has wider relevance.

[51] The methodology employed for this study refers to factors, practices, approaches, contextual features and so on as 'conditions'.

[52] Assessments were made for the time of completion and for three years previously. Asking respondents to make self-assessments for longer ago than three years was regarded as unreliable and likely to have too many non-responses due to staff turnover. See Chapter Three for further details of the assessment tools.

[53] 2009 for teenage conceptions.

[54] For female life expectancy a marginally significant difference was found.

[55] A table showing configurations of all the conditions in a QCA and their logical consequences regarding some outcome.

[56] The discussion of the results for cancers and CVD draws heavily on a paper by Blackman et al (2011).

[57] The discussion of the results for teenage conceptions draws heavily on a paper by Blackman et al (2013).

[58] I.e. what combinations of practice and context are associated with most progress towards the health inequality targets?

[59] Absolute gaps can be defined as the 'difference in performance between the disadvantaged and reference group' and relative gaps as the 'performance in the disadvantaged group as a proportion of performance in the reference group' (DH, 2008).

[60] Crouch (2000) raises some interesting issues about the extent of political debate in what he terms 'post-democracy' in advanced capitalist and neoliberal societies like the UK. This is beyond the scope of the discussion here, but Crouch's main argument is that political power, like income, is concentrated among elites, and the rest of us have very little say in the nature or direction of policy, thereby undermining the notion of a social contract acting as an arbiter of the 'general will' of the population.

References

Abbott, A, 2001, *Time matters*, Chicago: Chicago University Press

ACEVO, 2011, *Powerful people, responsible society, the report of the Commission on Big Society*, London: ACEVO

Acheson, D, 1998, *Independent enquiry into inequalities in health*, London: The Stationery Office

Ali, A, Wright, N and Rae, M, 2008, *Addressing health inequalities: A guide for general practitioners*, London: Royal College of General Practitioners

Allen, J, 2013, The Marmot public health review: how much progress has been made?, *The Guardian*, available at: www.theguardian.com/healthcare-network/2013/feb/01/marmot-review-progress-made

AMION Consulting, 2010, *Evaluation of the national strategy for neighbourhood renewal*, London: DCLG

Appleby, J, Ham, C, Imison, C and Jennings, M, 2010, *Improving NHS productivity: More with the same not more of the same*, London: The King's Fund

Association of Public Health Observatories, 2007, *Spearhead health inequalities intervention tool: Technical document*, London: APHO

Asthana, S and Halliday, J, 2006, *What works in tackling health inequalities?* Bristol: Policy Press

Atkinson, A B, 1970, On the measurement of inequality, *Journal of Economic Theory*, 2, 3, 244–63

Atkinson, R, Thomson, H, Kearns, A and Petticrew, M, 2006, Giving urban policy its 'medical': Assessing the place of health in area-based regeneration, *Policy & Politics*, 34, 1, 5–26

Australian Public Service Commission, 2007, *Tackling wicked problems: A public policy perspective*, Canberra: Australian Government

Baggott, R, 2004, *Health and health care in Britain*, Basingstoke: Palgrave Macmillan

Ball, M and Maginn, P J, 2004, The contradictions of urban policy: The case of the Single Regeneration Budget in London, *Environment and Planning C*, 22, 739–65

Ballard, D J, Nicewander, D A, Qin, H, Fullerton, C, Winter, F D and Couch, C E, 2007, Improving delivery of clinical preventive services: A multi-year journey, *American Journal of Preventive Medicine*, 33, 492–7

Bambra, C, 2012, Reducing health inequalities: New data suggest that the English strategy was partially successful, *Journal of Epidemiology and Public Health*, 66, 662

Bambra, C, Smith, K E, Garthwaite, K, Joyce, K and Hunter, D, 2011, A labour of Sisyphus? Public policy and health inequalities research from the Black and Acheson Reports to the Marmot Review, *Journal of Epidemiology and Community Health*, 65, 5, 399–406

Barber, M, 2008, *Instruction to deliver: Fighting to transform Britain's public services*, London: Methuen

Barnes, M, Matka, E and Sullivan, H, 2003, Evidence, understanding and complexity: Evaluation in non-linear systems, *Evaluation*, 9, 3, 265–84

Barr, B, Taylor-Robinson, D and Whitehead, M, 2012, Impact on health inequalities of rising prosperity in England 1998–2007, and implications for performance incentives: Longitudinal ecological study, *British Medical Journal*, 345, bmj.e5142

Barton, A, 1955, The concept of property space in social research, in Lazarsfeld, P and Rosenberg, M (eds), *The language of social research*, Glencoe: Free Press, 40–53

Baum, F, 2007, Cracking the nut of health equity: Top down and bottom up pressure for action on the social determinants of health, *Promotion & Education*, 14, 2, 90–5

Bennett, A and Elman, C, 2006, Complex causal relations and case study methods: The example of path dependence, *Political Analysis*, 14, 250–67

Bentley, C, 2008, *Systematically addressing health inequalities*, London: DH

Berg-Schlosser, D, and De Meur, G, 2009, Comparative research design: Case and variable selection, in Rihoux B and Ragin C (eds) *Configurational Comparative Method: Qualitative Comparative Analysis (QCA) and Related Techniques*, Los Angeles: SAGE Publications, Inc, 19–32

Berg-Schlosser, D, De Meur, G, Rihoux, B and Ragin, C, 2009, Qualitative comparative analysis (QCA) as an approach, in Rihoux, B and Ragin, C (eds), *Configurational comparative method: Qualitative comparative analysis (QCA) and related techniques*, Los Angeles: SAGE Publications, 1–18

Berridge, V, 2007, Multidisciplinary public health: What sort of victory? *Public Health*, 121, 404–08

Bevan, G and Hood, C, 2006, What's measured is what matters: Targets and gaming in the English public health care system, *Public Administration*, 84, 3, 517–38

Beveridge W, 1942, *Social Insurance and Allied Services*, cmd 6404, London: HMSO

Bhaskar, R, 1997, On the ontological status of ideas, *Journal of Theory of Social Behavior*, 27, 2–3, 139–47

Bivikar, R, 2011, *An exploration of the experience of patients who have had an episode of Tuberculosis in Bangladesh focusing on delay in seeking treatment and the socioeconomic impact on patients and their families*, PhD Thesis, Durham University

References

Black, D, 1980, *Inequalities in health*, London: DHSS

Blackman, T, 2006, *Placing health: Neighbourhood renewal, health improvement and complexity*, Bristol: Policy Press

Blackman, T and Dunstan, K, 2010, Qualitative comparative analysis and health inequalities: Investigating reasons for differential progress with narrowing local gaps in mortality, *Journal of Social Policy*, 39, 3, 359–73

Blackman, T, Harrington, B, Elliott, E, Greene, A, Hunter, D, Marks, L, McKee, L and Williams, G, 2006, Performance assessment and wicked issues: The case of health inequalities, *Public Policy and Administration*, 21, 2, 66–80

Blackman, T, Harrington, B, Elliott, E, Greene, A, Hunter, D, Marks, L, McKee, L and Williams, G, 2009, Tackling health inequalities in post-devolution Britain: Do targets matter?, *Public Administration*, 87, 762–78

Blackman, T, Hunter, D, Marks, L, Harrington, B, Elliott, E, Williams, G, Greene, A and Mckee, L, 2010, Wicked comparisons: Reflections on cross-national research about health inequalities in the UK, *Evaluation*, 16, 1, 43–57

Blackman, T, Wistow, J and Byrne, D, 2011a, A qualitative comparative analysis of factors associated with trends in narrowing health inequalities in England, *Social Science & Medicine*, 72, 12, 1965–74

Blackman, T, Wistow, J and Byrne, D, 2011b, *Towards a new understanding of how local action can effectively address health inequalities*, Report for the National Institute for Health Research Service Delivery and Organisation Programme, Project Ref: 08/1716/203

Blackman, T, Wistow, J and Byrne, D, 2013, Using qualitative comparative analysis to understand complex policy problems, *Evaluation*, 19, 2, 126–40

Blanden, J, Gregg, P and Machin, S, 2005, *Intergenerational mobility in Europe and North America*, Centre for Economic Performance, available at: http://cep.lse.ac.uk/about/news/IntergenerationalMobility.pdf

Blane, D, 1991, Inequality and social class, in Scambler, G (ed), *Sociology as applied to medicine*, London: Bailliere Tindall, 109–28

Bourdieu, P, 1986, The forms of capital, in Richardson, J (ed), *Handbook of Theory and Research for the Sociology of Education*, New York: Greenwood, 241–58

Bovaird, T, Willis, M and Briggs, I, 2014, Strategic commissioning for local public services: Service improvement cycle or just going round in circles?, *Local Government Studies*, 40, 4, 533–59

Brigden, P, 2006, Social capital, community empowerment and public health: Policy developments in the UK since 1997, *Policy and Politics*, 34, 27–50

Buck, D and Frosini, F, 2012, *Clustering of unhealthy behaviours over time: Implications for policy and practice*, London: King's Fund

Buck, D and Gregory, S, 2013, *Improving the public's health: A resource for local authorities*, London: King's Fund

Buijs, J-M, Echuis, J and Byrne, D, 2009, Approaches to researching complexity in public management, in Teisman, G, van Buren, A and Gerrits, L (eds), *Managing complex governance systems: Dynamics, self-organization and coevolution in public investments*, New York/London: Routledge, 37–55

Burawoy, M, 2005, For public sociology, *American Sociological Review*, 70, 1, 4–28

Buser, M, 2013, Tracing the democratic narrative: Big Society, localism and civic engagement, *Local Government Studies*, 39, 1, 3–21

Byrne, D, 1998, *Complexity theory and the social sciences*, London: Routledge

Byrne, D, 2002, *Interpreting quantitative data*, London: Sage

Byrne, D, 2005, *Social exclusion*, Maidenhead: Open University Press

Byrne, D, 2009, Complex realist and configurational approaches to cases: A radical synthesis, in Byrne, D and Ragin, C (eds), *The Sage handbook of case based methods*, London: Sage, 101–12

Byrne, D, 2011, *Applying social science: The role of social research in politics, policy and practice*, Bristol: Policy Press

Byrne, D, 2012, UK sociology and quantitative methods: Are we as weak as they think? Or are they barking up the wrong tree?, *Sociology*, 46, 1, 13–24

Byrne, D and Callaghan, G, 2013, *Complexity theory and the social sciences: The state of the art*, London: Routledge

Byrne, D, Olsen, W K and Duggan, S, 2009, Causality and interpretation in qualitative policy related research, in Byrne, D and Ragin, C (eds), *The Sage handbook of case based methods*, London: Sage, 511–21

Cabinet Office, 2010a, *The Coalition: Our programme for government*, London: Cabinet Office

Cabinet Office, 2010b, *Building the Big Society*, London: Cabinet Office

Callaghan, G, 2008, Evaluation and negotiated order: Developing the application of complexity theory, *Evaluation*, 14, 4, 393–405

Campbell, D, 2014, John Ashton: 'Inequality is our greatest challenge', *The Guardian*, 1 July 2014

Care Quality Commission, 2009, *Closing the gap: Tackling cardiovascular disease and health inequalities by prescribing statins and stop smoking services*, London: Care Quality Commission

Carr-Hill, R and Chalmers-Dixon, P, 2005, *The Public Health Observatory handbook of health inequalities measurement*, Oxford: South East Public Health Observatory

Cartwright, N, 2007a, Are RCTs the gold standard?, *BioSocieties*, 2, 11–20

Cartwright, N, 2007b, *Hunting causes and using them*, Cambridge: Cambridge University Press

Castellani, B and Castellani, J, 2003, Data mining: Qualitative analysis with health informatics data, *Qualitative Health Research*, 13, 1005–18

Castellani, B, Rajaram, R, Buckwalter, J G, Ball, M and Hafferty, F, 2012, Place and health as complex systems: A case study and empirical test, *Proceedings of the Center for Complexity in Health, Kent State University at Ashtabula*, 1, 1, 1–35

Castelli, A, Jacobs, R, Goddard, M and Smith, P, 2013, Health, policy and geography: Insights from a multi-level modelling approach, *Social Science and Medicine*, 92, 61–73

Chadwick, E, 1842, *Report from the Poor Law Commissioners on an Inquiry into the Sanitary Conditions of the Labouring Population of Great Britain*, London: Poor Law Commission

Chapman, J, 2004, *System failure: Why governments must learn to think differently*, London: Demos

Checkland, K, Allen, P, Coleman, A, Segar, J, McDermott, I, Harrison, S, Petsoulas, C and Peckham, S, 2013, Accountable to whom, for what? An exploration of the early development of clinical commissioning groups in the English NHS, *British Medical Journal*, 3:e003769.doi:10.1136/bmjopen-2013-003769

Cilliers, P, 1998, *Complexity and postmodernism*, London: Routledge

Cilliers, P, 2001, Boundaries, hierarchies and networks in complex systems, *International Journal of Innovation Management*, 5, 2, 135–47

Cilliers, P, 2008, Paul Cilliers, in Gershenson, C. (ed), *Complexity: 5 questions*, Copenhagen: Automatic Press/VIP, 43–50

Clark, T, 2014, How the Tories chose to hit the poor, *The Guardian*, 2nd July 2014, available at: www.theguardian.com/commentisfree/2014/jul/02/tories-poor-george-osborne-inequality-conservatives

Clark, W R, Gilligan, M J and Golder, M, 2006, A simple multivariate test for asymmetric hypotheses, *Political Analysis*, 14, 311–31

Clarke, J, 2006, Scrutiny through inspection and audit: Policies, structures and processes, in Budd, L J, Charlesworth, J and Paton, R (eds), *Making policy happen*, London: Routledge, 205–15

Clarke, J and Newman, J, 2012, The alchemy of austerity, *Critical Social Policy*, 32, 3, 299–319

Coates, D, 2010, Keeping the Tories at bay, *Renewal*, 18, 1/2, 113–21

Cochrane, A L, 1972, *Effectiveness and efficiency: Random reflections on health services*, London: Nuffield Provincial Hospitals Trust

Cohn, S, Clinch, M, Bunn, C and Stronge, P, 2013, Entangled complexity: why complex interventions are just not complicated enough, *Journal of Health Services Research & Policy*, 18, 1, 40–3

Coleman, A, Checkland, K, Segar, J, McDermott, I, Harrison, S and Peckham, S, 2014, Joining it up? Health and wellbeing boards in English local governance: Evidence from clinical commissioning groups and shadow health and wellbeing boards, *Local Government Studies*, 40, 4, 560–80

Coleman, L, 2002, New opportunities for reducing the risk from teenage pregnancy: What is the evidence base for tackling risk behaviours in combination?, *Health, Risk and Society*, 4, 1, 77–93

Collinge, A, Duffy, B and Page, B, 2005, *Physical capital: Liveability in 2005*, London: MORI

Commission on Social Justice, 1994, *Social justice, strategies for national renewal: Report of the Commission on Social Justice*, London: Vintage

Cooper, B, 2005, Applying Ragin's crisp and fuzzy set QCA to large datasets: Social class and educational achievement in the NCDS, *Sociological Research Online*, available at: www.socresonline.org.uk/10/2/cooper1.html

Corbett, S and Walker, A, 2013, The Big Society: Rediscovery of the social or rhetorical fig-leaf for neo-liberalism, *Critical Social Policy*, 33, 3, 451–72

Craig, J, 2013, *Reducing health inequalities: The challenge of public health*, London: British Council

Cribb, J, Hood, A, Joyce, R and Phillips, D, 2013, *Living standards, poverty and inequality in the UK: 2013*, London: Institute for Fiscal Studies

Cropper, S, 2002, What contribution might ideas of social capital make to policy implementation for reducing health inequalities?, Paper in HDA Seminar Series 'Tackling health inequalities: Turning policy into practice'

Crouch, C, 2000, *Coping with post democracy*, London: The Fabian Society

Crouch, C, 2011, *The strange non-death of neo-liberalism*, Cambridge: Polity Press

Cummins, S, Curtis, S E, Diez-Roux, A V and Macintyre, S, 2007, Understanding and representing 'place' in health research: A relational approach, *Social Science & Medicine*, 66, 2, 1825–38

Curtis, S, 2008, How can we address health inequality through healthy public policy in Europe?, *European Urban and Regional Studies*, 15, 4, 293–305

Dahlgren, G and Whitehead, M, 1991, *Policies and strategies to promote social equity in health*, Stockholm: Institute for Future Studies

Davis, P, West, K and Yardley, L, 2011, Networks in open systems of governance, *Public Management Review*, 13, 5, 683–705

Dawson, M, 2013, Against the Big Society: a Durkheimian socialist critique, *Critical Social Policy*, 33, 1, 78–96

DCLG (Department for Communities and Local Government), 2007, *Common themes: Local strategic partnerships and teenage pregnancy*, London: DCLG

DCSF/DH (Department for Children, Schools and Families/Department of Health), 2010, *Teenage pregnancy strategy: Beyond 2010*, London: DCSF Publications

Department for Education and Skills, 2006a, *Teenage pregnancy: Accelerating the strategy to 2010*, Nottingham: Department for Education and Skills

Department for Education and Skills, 2006b, *Teenage pregnancy next steps: Guidance for local authorities and primary care trusts on effective delivery of local strategies*, Nottingham: Department for Education and Skills

DH, 1999, *National service framework for mental health: Modern standards and service models*, London: DH

DH, 2000a, *Coronary heart disease: National service framework for coronary heart disease – modern standards and service models*, London: DH

DH, 2000b, *The NHS cancer plan: A plan for investment, a plan for reform*, London: DH

DH, 2002, *Tackling health inequalities: A cross-cutting review*, London: DH

DH, 2003, *Tackling health inequalities: A programme for action*, London: DH

DH, 2004a, *Tackling health inequalities: The Spearhead group of local authorities and primary care trusts*, London: DH

DH, 2004b, *Choosing health*, London: DH

DH, 2005, *Tackling health inequalities: What works*, London: DH

DH, 2006, *Tackling health inequalities: 2003–05 data update for the national 2010 PSA target*, London: DH

DH, 2007a, *Tackling health inequalities: 2004–06 data and policy update for the 2010 national target*, London: DH

DH, 2007b, *Commissioning framework for health and well-being*, London: DH

DH, 2007c, *World class commissioning: Vision*, London: DH

DH, 2007d, *Tackling health inequalities: Programme for action*, London: DH

DH, 2008, *Tackling health inequalities: 2007 status report on the programme for action*, London: DH

DH, 2009, *Tackling health inequalities: 10 years on*, London: DH

DH, 2010a, *NHS outcomes framework 2011/2012*, London: CIO

DH, 2010b, *Equity and excellence: Liberating the NHS*, London: The Stationery Office

DH, 2011, *Public health in local authorities: Commissioning responsibilities*, London: DH

DH, 2012, *Healthy lives, healthy people: Improving outcomes and supporting transparency*, London: DH

DH, 2013, *The Mandate: A mandate from the government to the NHS Commissioning Board: April 2013 to March 2015*, London: DH

DH and DCLG, 2010, *Liberating the NHS: Local democratic legitimacy in health*, London: DH and DCLG

DHSS (Department of Health and Social Security), 1976, *Prevention and health: Everybody's business*, London: HMSO.

DHSS, 1977, *Prevention and health*, London: HMSO

DHSS, 1987, *Promoting better health*, London: HMSO

Dixon, A, Khachatryan, A, Wallace, A, Peckham, S, Boyce, T and Gillam, S, 2011, *Impact of quality and outcomes framework on health inequalities*, London: King's Fund

Dixon-Woods, M, Bonas, S, Booth, A, Jones, D, Miller, T, Sutton, A, Shaw, R, Smith, J and Young, B, 2006, How can systematic reviews incorporate qualitative research? A critical perspective, *Qualitative Research*, 6, 27–44

Doetter, L and Gotze, R, 2011, Health care policy for better or for worse? Examining NHS Reforms During Times of Economic Crisis versus Relative Stability, *Social Policy and Administration*, 45, 4, 488–505

Dorling, D, 2011, *Injustice: Why social inequality persists*, Bristol: Policy Press

Dorling, D, 2013a, *Unequal health: The scandal of our times*, Bristol: Policy Press

Dorling, D, 2013b, *In place of fear: Narrowing health inequalities*, London: Centre for Labour and Social Studies

Dyer, W, 2006, The psychiatric and criminal careers of mentally disordered offenders referred to a custody diversion team in the United Kingdom, *International Journal of Forensic Mental Health*, 5, 1, 15–28

Erreygers, G, 2013, Dual Atkinson measure of socioeconomic inequality of health, *Health Economics*, 22, 4, 466–79

Evans, D, 2011, The Big Society needs robust public health evaluation, *Journal of Public Health*, 33, 1, 11–12

Exworthy, M and Powell, M, 2004, Big windows and little windows: Implementation in the 'congested state', *Public Administration*, 82, 2, 263–81

Ferragina, E, 2010, Social capital and equality: Tocqueville's legacy: Rethinking social capital in relation with income inequalities, *The Tocqueville Review*, 31, 1, 73–98

Finlayson, A, 2010, The broken society versus the social recession, *Soundings*, 44, 22–34

Fiss, P, 2007, A set-theoretic approach to organizational configurations, *Academy of Management Review*, 32, 1180–98

Fiss, P, 2009, Case studies and the configurational analysis of organizational phenomena, in Byrne, D and Ragin, C (eds), *Sage handbook of case based research*, London: Sage, 424–40

Fotaki, M, 2007, Can directors of public health implement the new public health agenda in primary care? A case study of primary care trusts in the north west of England, *Policy and Politics*, 35, 311–35

French, R, Joyce, L, Fenton, K, Kingori, P, Griffiths, C, Stone, V, Patel-Kanwal, H, Power, R, and Stephenson, J, 2005, *Exploring the attitudes and behaviours of Bangladeshi, Indian and Jamaican young people in relation to reproductive and sexual health*, London: Teenage Pregnancy Unit

Gerrits, L, 2008, *The gentle art of coevolution: A complexity theory perspective on decision making over estuaries in Germany, Belgium and the Netherlands*, Rotterdam: Erasmus Universiteit

Glaesser, J, Gott, R, Roberts, R and Cooper, B, 2009a, The roles of substantive and procedural understanding in open-ended science investigations: Using fuzzy set qualitative comparative analysis to compare two different tasks, *Research in Science Education*, 39, 595–624

Glaesser, J, Gott, R, Roberts, R and Cooper, B, 2009b, Underlying success in open-ended investigations in science: Using qualitative comparative analysis to identify necessary and sufficient conditions, *Research in Science & Technological Education*, 27, 1, 5–30

Glasby, J, 2012, *Understanding health and social care*, Bristol: Policy Press

Glasman, M, 2010, Society not state: The challenge of the Big Society, *Public Policy Research*, 17, 2, 59–63

Goldstein, H, 2010, *Multilevel statistical models* (4th edn), London: Wiley-Blackwell

Goldthorpe, J and Jackson, M, 2007, Intergenerational class mobility in contemporary Britain: Political concerns and empirical findings, *The British Journal of Sociology*, 58, 4, 525–46

Goodley, S and Inman, P, 2013, Zero-hours contracts cover more than 1m UK workers, *The Guardian*, 5 August 2013

Graham, H, 2004, Tackling inequalities in health in England: Remedying health disadvantages, narrowing health gaps or reducing health gradients?, *Journal of Social Policy*, 33, 1, 115–31

Graham, H and Kelly, M P, 2004, *Health inequalities: Concepts, frameworks and policy*, London: Health Development Agency

Green, M, 2013, The equalisation hypothesis and changes in geographical inequalities of age based mortality in England, 2002–2004 to 2008–2010, *Social Sciences and Medicine*, 87, 93–8

Greenhalgh, T, 2009, Complexity theory and family medicine: A new symbiosis, *Swiss Journal of Family Medicine*, 331, 1

Gregory, S, Dixon, A and Ham, C, 2012, *Health policy under the coalition government: A mid-term assessment*, London: The King's Fund

Griffin, D (ed), 2006, *Complexity and the experience of managing in public sector organizations*, Abingdon: Routledge

Grimshaw, D and Rubery, J, 2012, The end of the UK's liberal collectivist social model? The implications of the coalition government's policy during the austerity crisis, *Cambridge Journal of Economics*, 36, 1, 105–26

Grint, K, 2008, Wicked problems and clumsy solutions: The role of leadership, *Clinical Leader*, 1, 2

Grofman, B and Schneider, C C, 2009, An introduction to crisp set QCA, with a comparison to binary logistic regression, *Political Research Quarterly*, 62, 662–72

Ham, C, 2014, *The NHS five year forward view: The man matters more than the plan*, London: The King's Fund

Hamlin, C and Sheard, S, 1998, Revolutions in public health: 1848, and 1998, *British Medical Journal*, 317, 7158, 587–91

Hancock, L and Mooney, G, 2013, 'Welfare ghettos' and the 'broken society': Territorial stigmatisation in the contemporary UK, *Housing, Theory and Society*, 30, 1, 46–64

Haynes, P, 2008, Complexity theory and evaluation in public management: A qualitative systems approach, *Public Management Review*, 10, 3, 401–19

Head, B, 2007, Three lenses of evidence-based policy, *Australian Journal of Public Administration*, 67, 1–11

Helm, T, 2014, The NHS is out of control, says Tory health minister, *The Guardian*, 21 June 2014, www.theguardian.com/society/2014/jun/21/nhs-control-given-away-tory-minister

HM Government, 2010a, *Decentralisation and the Localism Bill: an essential guide*, London: DCLG

HM Government, 2010b, *Healthy lives, healthy people: Our strategy for public health in England*, London: The Stationery Office

HM Treasury, 2004, *Spending review: Stability, security and opportunity for all: Investing for Britain's long-term future*, London: HM Treasury

House of Commons Health Committee, 2009, *Health inequalities: Third report of session 2008–2009*, London: The Stationery Office

House of Commons Health Committee, 2012, *Social care: Fourteenth report of session 2010–12, Volume I: Report, together with formal minutes*, London: The Stationery Office

House of Commons Health Committee, 2014, *Public Health England: Eighth report of session 2013–14*, London: The Stationery Office

Humphries, R and Galea, A, 2013, *Health and wellbeing boards: One year on*, London: The King's Fund

Hunter, D and Killoran, A, 2004, *Tackling health inequalities: Turning policy into practice?*, London: Health Development Agency

Hunter, D, Marks, L and Smith K, 2007, *The public health system in England: A scoping study*, London: National Institute for Health Research Service Delivery and Organisation

Hunter, D, Marks, L and Smith, K, 2010, *The public health system in England*, Bristol: Policy Press

Hutton, W, 2003, *The world we're in*, London: Abacus

IFS, 2014, *The IFS Green Budget: February 2014*, London: Institute for Fiscal Studies

Iles, V and Sutherland, K, 2001, *Organisational change: A review for health care managers, professionals and researchers*, London: National Coordinating Centre for the Service Delivery and Organisation

Illich, I, 1975, *Medical nemesis: The expropriation of health*, New York: Pantheon Books

Illich, I, 1976, *Limits to medicine, medical nemesis: The expropriation of health*, London: Marion Boyars

Introna, L, 2003, Complexity theory and organisational intervention? Dealing with (in)commensurability, in Mittleton-Kelly, E (ed), *Complex systems and evolutionary perspectives on organisations*, Oxford: Pergamon, 205–20

Ismail, S, Thorlby, R and Holder, H, 2014, *Focus on: Social care for older people*, London: The Health Foundation and Nuffield Trust

Järvinen, Y L N, Sievänen, H, Kannus, P, Jokihaara, J and Khan, K M, 2011, The true cost of pharmacological disease prevention, *British Medical Journal*, 342, d2175

Kamarck, E C, 2007, *The end of government ... as we know it*, London: Lynne Rienner Publications

Kathol, R G, Butler, M, McAlpine, D D and Kane, R L, 2010, Barriers to physical and mental condition integrated service delivery, *Psychosomatic Medicine*, 72, 511–8

Kelly, M, 2010, The axes of social differentiation and the evidence base on health equity, *Journal of the Royal Society of Medicine*, 103, 7, 266–72

Kintrea, K and Morgan, J, 2005, *Evaluation of English housing policy 1975–2000*, London: Office of the Deputy Prime Minister

Klein, R, 1995, *The new politics of the NHS*, Harlow: Pearson Education Limited

Klijn, E H, 2008, Governance and governance networks in Europe: An assessment of 10 years of research on the theme, *Public Management Review*, 10, 4, 505–25

Klijn, E H and Snellen, I T M, 2009, Complexity theory and public administration: A critical appraisal, in Teisman, G, van Buren, M and Gerrits, L (eds), *Managing complex governance systems: Dynamics, self-organization and coevolution in public investments*, London: Routledge, 17–36

Knapp, M, Hardy, B and Forder, J, 2001, Commissioning for quality: Ten years of social care markets in England, *Journal of Social Policy*, 30, 2, 283–306

Kooiman, J, 2003, *Governing as governance*, London: Sage

Lakin, M, 2013, The ideology of the coalition: More muscular then liberal?' *British Politics*, 8, 476–90

Lazarsfeld, P, 1937, Some remarks on typological procedures in social research, *Zeitschrift Fur Sozialforschung*, 6, 119–39

Lee, N, Sissons, P and Jones, K, 2013, *Wage inequality and employment polarisation in British cities*. London: The Work Foundation

Lieberson, S, 1985, *Making it count*, Berkeley: California University Press

Longest, K and Vaisey, S, 2008, Fuzzy: A program for performing qualitative comparative analyses (QCA) in Stata, *STATA Journal*, 8, 3–28

Lowndes, V and Pratchett, L, 2012, Local governance under the coalition government: Austerity, localism and the 'Big Society', *Local Government Studies*, 38, 1, 1–20

Lupton, R and Power, A, 2002, Social exclusion and neighbourhoods, in Hills, J and Le Grand, J (eds), *Understanding social exclusion*, Oxford: Oxford University Press, 118–40

Lupton, R, with Hills, J, Stewart, K and Vizard, P, 2013, *Labour's social policy record: Policy, spending and outcomes 1997–2010*, London: Centre for Analysis of Social Exclusion

MacIntosh, R, MacLean, D, Stacey, R and Griffin, D (eds), 2006, *Complexity and organization: Readings and conversations*, London: Routledge

MacIver, R M, 1942, *Social causation*, New York: Ginn and Company

Mackenbach, J P, 2010, Has the English strategy to reduce health inequalities failed?, *Social Science and Medicine*, 71, 7, 1249–53

Mackenbach, J P, 2011, Can we reduce health inequalities? An analysis of the English strategy, *Journal of Epidemiology and Community Health*, 65, 568–75

Marmot, M, 2004, *Status syndrome*, London: Bloomsbury

Marmot, M, 2010, *Fair society, healthy lives: Strategic review of health inequalities in England post-2010*, London: The Marmot Review

Marmot, M, 2014, Foreword, in *If you could do one thing … Nine local actions to reduce health inequalities*, London: British Academy, 6–7

Matheson, A, Dew, K and Cumming, J, 2009, Complexity, evaluation, and the effectiveness of community-based interventions to reduce health inequalities, *Health Promotion Journal of Australia*, 20, 3, 221–6

McKeown, T, 1976, *The role of medicine: Dream, mirage or nemesis?* London: Nuffield Provincial Hospitals Trust

Meadows, D H, 2009, *Thinking in systems: A primer*, London: Earthscan

Meehl, P M, 1970, Nuisance variables and the ex post facto design, in Radner, M and Winokur, S (eds), *Minnesota studies in the philosophy of science: IV.* Minneapolis: University of Minnesota, 373–402

Miller, R, Peckham, S, Checkland, K, Coleman, A, McDermott, I, Harrison, S, and Segar, J, 2012, *Clinical engagement in primary care-led commissioning: A review of the evidence*, London: Policy Research Unit in Commissioning and the Healthcare System

Milligan, C, 2009, *There's no place like home: Place and care in an ageing society*, Aldershot, Ashgate

Mills, C W, 1962, *The sociological imagination*, New York: Oxford University Press

Mitchell, M, 2011, *Complexity: A guided tour*, Oxford: Oxford University Press

Morgan, S and Winship, C, 2007, *Counterfactuals and causal inference*, Cambridge: Cambridge University Press

MRC (Medical Research Council) (2000) *A framework for the development and evaluation of RCTs for complex interventions to improve health*, London: MRC

MRC (2008) *Developing and evaluating complex interventions: New guidance*, London: MRC

Murray, C, 1984, *Losing ground: American social policy 1950–1980*, New York: Basic Books

NAO (National Audit Office), 2010, *Tackling inequalities in life expectancy in areas with the worst health and deprivation*, London: The Stationery Office

NAO, 2013, *Early action: Landscape review*, London: The Stationery Office

National Cancer Inequality Initiative, 2010, *Reducing cancer inequality: Evidence, progress and making it happen*, London: DH

Nathanson, C, 2007, *Disease prevention as social change: The state, society, and public health in the United States, France, Great Britain, and Canada*, New York: Russell Sage Foundation

Nathanson, C, 2010, Who owns health inequalities?, *The Lancet*, 375, 9711, 274–5

Nathanson, C and Hopper, K, 2010, The Marmot Review: Social revolution by stealth, *Social Sciences and Medicine*, 71, 1237–9

National Equality Panel, 2010, *An anatomy of economic inequality in the UK*, London: Centre for Analysis of Social Exclusion

NHS, 2000, *National Cancer Plan*, London: DH

NHS, 2014, *Five year forward view*, London: NHS

NICE (National Institute for Health and Care Excellence), 2008, *NICE public health guidance 10: Smoking cessation services: Implementation advice*. London: NICE

Nutley, S M, Walter, I and Davies, H T O, 2007, *Using evidence: How research can inform public services*, Bristol: Policy Press

Oliver, A, 2008, *Reflections on the development of health inequalities policy in the United Kingdom*, London: LSE Health working papers

Oliver, M, 1990, *The individual and social models of disability*, Paper presented at Joint Workshop of the Living Options Group and the Research Unit of the Royal College of Physicians

Olsen, W and Nomura, H, 2009, Poverty reduction: Fuzzy sets vs. crisp sets compared, *Sociological Theory and Method*, 24, 218–46

ONS (Office for National Statistics), 2013a, *Labour market statistics, September 2013*, London: ONS

ONS, 2013b, *Estimating zero-hour contracts from the labour force survey*, London: ONS

ONS, 2014a, *Healthy life expectancy at birth for upper tier local authorities: England, 2010–12*, London: ONS

ONS, 2014b, *June labour market statistics*, London: ONS, www.ons.gov.uk/ons/dcp171778_363998.pdf

Pantazis, C and Gordon, D (eds), 2000, *Tackling health inequalities: Where are we now and what can be done?*, Bristol: Policy Press

Parliament, 1979, *Royal Commission on the NHS*, Cmnd 7615, London: HMSO

Pawson, R and Tilley, N, 1997, *Realistic evaluation*, London: Sage

Pearce, J, 2012, The 'blemish of place': stigma, geography and health inequalities, *Social Science and Medicine*, 75, 1921–4

Pearce, J, 2013, Financial crisis, austerity policies and geographical inequalities in health, *Environment and Planning A*, 45, 2030–45

Peckham, S and Exworthy, M, 2003, *Primary care in the UK: Policy, organisation and management*, Basingstoke: Palgrave Macmillan

Petticrew, M and Roberts, H, 2003, Evidence, hierarchies, and typologies: Horses for courses, *Journal of Epidemiology and Community Health*, 57, 527–9

Petticrew, M, Tugwell, P, Welch, V, Ueffing, E, Kristjansson, E, Armstrong, R, Doyle, J and Waters, E, 2009, Cochrane update: Better evidence about wicked issues in tackling health inequalities, *Journal of Public Health*, 31, 3, 453–6

PHE (Public Health England), 2014a, *Heatwave plan for England*, London: PHE

PHE, 2014b, *From evidence into action: Opportunities to protect and improve the nation's health*, London: PHE

Plsek, P, 2001, Redesigning health care with insights from the science of complex adaptive systems, in *Crossing the quality chasm: A new health system for the 21st century*, Washington DC: National Academy Press, 309–322

Pollock, A, Price, D, Roderick, P, Treuherz, T, McCoy, D, McKee, M and Reynolds, L, 2012, How the Health and Social Care Bill 2011 would end entitlement to comprehensive health care in England, *The Lancet*, 379, 9814, 387–9

Porter, S, 2013, Capitalism, the state and health care in the age of austerity: A Marxist analysis, *Nursing Philosophy*, 14, 1, 5–16

Public Accounts Committee, 2013, *Department for Communities and Local Government: Financial sustainability of local authorities*, London: The Stationery Office

Putman, R, 1995, Bowling alone: America's declining social capital, *Journal of Democracy*, 6, 1, 65–78

Ragin, C, 1987, *The comparative method*, Berkeley: California University Press

Ragin, C, 1992, Casing and the process of social inquiry, in Becker and Ragin (eds), *What is a case?* Cambridge: Cambridge University Press, 217–26

Ragin, C, 2000, *Fuzzy set social science*, Chicago: Chicago University Press

Ragin, C, 2006a, The limitations of net effects thinking, in Rihoux, B and Grimm, H (eds), *Innovative comparative methods for political analysis*, New York: Springer, 13–41

Ragin, C, 2006b, Set relations in social research: Evaluating their consistency and coverage, *Political Analysis*, 14, 291–310

Ragin, C, 2008, *Redesigning social inquiry*, Chicago: Chicago University Press

Richards, M, 2007, *Cancer ten years on*, London: DH

Rihoux, B and De Meur, G, 2009, Crisp-set qualitative comparative analysis (csQCA), in Rihoux, B and Ragin, C (eds), *Configurational comparative method: Qualitative comparative analysis (QCA) and related techniques*, Los Angeles: SAGE Publications, 33–68

Rihoux, B and Lobe, B, 2009, The case for qualitative comparative analysis (QCA): Adding leverage for thick cross-case comparison, in Byrne, D and Ragin, C (eds), *Sage handbook of case based research*, London: Sage, 222–42

Rihoux, B and Ragin, C, 2009, Introduction, in Rihoux, B and Ragin, C (eds), *Configurational comparative method: Qualitative comparative analysis (QCA) and related techniques*, Los Angeles: SAGE Publications, xvii–xxv

Rittel, H and Webber, M, 1973, Dilemmas in a general theory of planning, *Policy Sciences*, 4, 155–69

Rosen, R, 1987, Some epistemological issues in physics and biology, in Hiley, B and Peat, F (eds), *Quantum implications: Essays in honour of David Bohm*, London: Routledge, 314–27

Rowlingson, K, 2011, *Does income inequality cause health and social problems?* York: Joseph Rowntree Foundation

Roy, B, 2012, *An exploration of the experience of patients who have had an episode of Tuberculosis in Bangladesh focusing on delay in seeking treatment and the socioeconomic impact on patients and their families*, Durham theses, Durham University, http://etheses.dur.ac.uk/4419/

RSPH (Royal Society for Public Health), 2014 *The RSPH guide to commissioning for health improvement*, London: Royal Society for Public Health

Sassi, F, 2005, Tackling health inequalities in a more equal society?, in Hills, J and Stewart, K (eds), *New Labour, poverty, inequality and exclusion*, Bristol: Policy Press, 69–92

Scally, G, 2013, *Have we lost the battle to improve health inequalities?* King's Fund Blog, 24 January 2013, www.kingsfund.org.uk/time-to-think-differently/blog/have-we-lost-battle-improve-health-inequalities

Scambler, G, 2011, 'Tackling health inequalities' and its pros, cons and contradictions: a commentary on Blackman, Wistow and Byrne, *Social Science and Medicine*, 72, 12, 1975–7

Seamark, C J and Gray, D J P, 1998, Teenagers and risk-taking: Pregnancy and smoking, *British Journal of General Practice*, 48, 985–6

Secretary of State for Health, 1998, *Our healthier nation*, London: HMSO

Secretary of State for Health, 1999, *Saving lives: Our healthier nation*, Cm 4386, London: HMSO

Seddon, J, 2005, *Freedom from command and control: A better way to make the work work*, Buckingham: Vanguard Education

Seddon, J, 2008, *Systems thinking in the public sector*, Axminster: Triarchy Press

Sefton, T and Sutherland, H, 2005, Inequality and poverty under New Labour, in Hills, J and Stewart, K (eds), *New Labour, poverty, inequality and exclusion*, Bristol: Policy Press, 231–50

Shaw, M and Dorling, D, 2004, Who cares in England and Wales? The positive care law, *British Journal of General Practice*, 54, 899–903

Shaw, M, Dorling, D, Gordon, D and Davey Smith, G, 1999, *The widening gap: health inequalities and policy in Britain*, Bristol: Policy Press

Smith, P C, 2005, Performance measurement in health care: History, challenges and prospects, *Public Money and Management*, 25, 213–20

Spinakis, A, Anastasiou, G, Panoussis, V, Spiliopoulos, K, Palaiologou, S and Yfantopoulos, J, 2011, *Expert review and proposals for measurement of health inequalities in the European Union: Full report*, Luxembourg: EU Directorate-General for Health and Consumers

Social Exclusion Unit, 2001, *A new commitment to neighbourhood renewal: National strategy action plan*, London: Cabinet Office

Staite, C and Miller, R, 2011, *Health and wellbeing boards: Developing a successful partnership*, Birmingham: INLOGOV and HSMC

Stocking, B, 1985, *Initiative and inertia: Case studies in the NHS*, London: The Nuffield Provincial Hospitals Trust

Stoker, G, 1998, Governance as theory: Five propositions, *International Social Science Journal*, 155, 17–28

Suckling, R, 2010, *Early lung cancer intervention in Doncaster: Doncaster 3 week cough: How to Guide*, London: Cancer Research UK, available at: http://info.cancerresearchuk.org/prod_consump/groups/cr_common//@nre/@hea/documents/generalcontent/cr_043172.pdf

Taylor, S and Marandi, A, 2008, Social determinants of health and the design of health programs for the poor, *British Medical Journal*, 332, a209

Taylor-Gooby, P, 2012, Root and branch restructuring to achieve major cuts: The social policy programme of the 2010 UK coalition government, *Social Policy & Administration*, 46, 1, 61–82

Teenage Pregnancy Unit, 2005, *East London papers: Appendix A: Literature review*, London: Department for Education

Teisman, G, Gerrits, L and van Buren, A, 2009, Understanding and managing complex process systems, in Teisman, G, van Buren, A and Gerrits, L (eds), *Managing complex governance systems: Dynamics, self-organization and coevolution in public investments*, New York/London: Routledge, 1–16

Thaler, R and Sunstein, C, 2008, *Nudge: Improving decisions about health, wealth, and happiness*, New Haven: Yale University Press

Timmins, N, 1995, *The five giants: A biography of the welfare state*, London: Fontana Press

Timmins, N, 2012, *Never again? The story of the Health and Social Care Act 2012*, London: The King's Fund

Townsend, P, Davidson, N and Whitehead, M (eds), 1992, *Inequalities in health: the Black Report and the health divide*, London: Penguin Books

Travers, M, 2007, *The new bureaucracy: Quality assurance and its critics*, Bristol: Policy Press

Tudor Hart, J, 1971, Inverse care law, *Lancet*, 1, 405–12

Tunstall, H, Mitchell, R, Gibbs, J, Platt, S and Dorling, D, 2007, Is economic adversity always a killer? Disadvantaged areas with relatively low mortality rates, *Journal of Epidemiology and Community Health*, 61, 337–43

Turner, D, Salway, S, Mir, G, Eillison, G, Skinner, J, Carter, L and Bostan, B, 2013, Prospects for progress on health inequalities in England in the post-primary care trust era: Professional views on challenges, risks and opportunities, *BMC Public Health*, 13, 274

Turner, R H, 1948, Statistical logic in social research, *Sociology and Social Research*, 32, 697–704

Uprichard, E and Byrne, D, 2006, Representing complex places: a narrative approach, *Environment and Planning A*, 38, 665–76

Uprichard, E and Byrne, D, 2007, Crossing levels, *Methodological Innovations Online*, 2, 1, 41–58

Vizard, P and Obolenskaya, P, 2013, *Labour's record on health*, London: Centre for Analysis of Social Exclusion

Wacquant, L, 2008, *Urban outcasts: A comparative sociology of advanced marginality*, Cambridge: Polity Press

Walby, S, Armstrong, J and Strid, S, 2012, Intersectionality: Multiple inequalities in social theory, *Sociology*, 46, 2, 224–40

Wallace, R and Wallace, D, 1997, Resilience and persistence of the synergism of plagues: Stochastic resonance and the ecology of disease, disorder and disinvestment in US urban neighborhoods, *Environment and Planning A*, 29, 789–804

Walsh, D, Whyte, B and Gordon, D S, 2007, Changing places? A comparative analysis of area-based health trends in Scotland through the 1980s and 1990s, *Public Health*, 121: 889–97

Wanless, D, 2004, *Securing good health for the whole population: Final report*, London: HM Treasury

Warr, D, Mann, R and Kelaher, M, 2013, A lot of the things we do … people wouldn't recognise as health promotion: Addressing health inequalities in settings of neighbourhood disadvantage, *Critical Public Health*, 23, 1, 95–109

Weber, M, 1947, *The Theory of Social and Economic Organization, translated by A.M. Henderson and Talcott Parsons. Edited with an introduction by Talcott Parsons*, New York: Free Press

Westergaard, J, 1978, Social policy and class inequality: some notes on welfare state limits, in Miliband, R and Saville, J (eds), *Socialist Register 1978*, London: Merlin Books, 71–99

Westergaard, J and Resler, H, 1975, *Class in a capitalist society: A study of contemporary Britain*, Harmondsworth: Pelican Books

Westrick, S C and Breland, M L, 2009, Sustainability of pharmacy-based innovations: The case of in-house immunization services, *Journal of the American Pharmacists Association*, 49, 500–508

Whitehead, M and Popay, J, 2010, Swimming upstream: Taking action on the social determinants of health inequalities, *Social Science and Medicine*, 71, 7, 1234–6

WHO (World Health Organization), 1948, Preamble to the Constitution of the World Health Organization as adopted by the International Health Conference, New York, 19–22 June, 1946; signed on 22 July 1946 by the representatives of 61 States, *Official Records of the World Health Organization*, 2, 100, and entered into force on 7 April 1948

WHO, 2008, *Closing the gap in a generation: Health equity through action on the social determinants of health*, Geneva: WHO

Wilkinson, R, 1976, Dear David Ennals, *New Society*, 16 December 1976, 567–8

Wilkinson, R and Pickett, K, 2010, *The spirit level: Why equality is better for everyone*, London: Penguin Books

Williams, R, 1980, Base and superstructure in Marxist cultural theory, in *Problems in materialism and culture: Selected essays*, London: Verso and NLB, 31–49

Wilson, W J, 1987, *The truly disadvantaged*, Chicago: University of Chicago Press

Wistow, G, 2011, Integration and the NHS reforms, *Journal of Integrated Care*, 19, 4, 5–13

Wistow, G, 2012, Still a fine mess? Local government and the NHS 1962 to 2012, *Journal of Integrated Care*, 20, 2, 101–14

Wistow, J, Dominelli, L, Oven, K, Dunn, C and Curtis, S, 2015, The role of formal and informal networks in supporting older people's care during extreme weather events, *Policy and Politics* (forthcoming)

Wrede, S, Benoit C, Bourgeault, I L, van Teijlingen, E R, Sandall, J and De Vries, R G, 2006, Decentred comparative research: Context sensitive analysis of maternal health care, *Social Science & Medicine*, 63, 11, 2986–97

Wright, R, 2001, *Nonzero: History, evolution and human cooperation*, London: Abacas

Zöllner, H, 2002, National policies for reducing social inequalities in health in Europe, *Scandinavian Journal of Public Health*, 30, 6–11

Practical techniques of the HINST approach

HINST has produced a raft of guides based on the effective practice it observed through the 70 visits it made to local teams. The practical lessons evolved into a consistent set of principles.

HINST produced a number of practical toolkits that are available on the HINST Associates website, in addition to those referenced above.[1] These include toolkits on:

- how to model the scale of use of evidence-based interventions necessary to reduce inequalities in life expectancy;
- how to develop and implement a balanced scorecard to tackle health inequalities through primary care;
- how to develop a taxonomy of general medical practices to support and encourage performance development;
- how to model need and develop a workforce plan to manage chronic disease registers as an industrial-scale process;
- achieving population health impact by systematically addressing the quality and cost–effectiveness of prescribing as part of the management of major killer chronic diseases in primary care;
- how to develop an ongoing programme of GP chronic disease management audits using a z-score-based dashboard;
- how to develop and implement a strategic framework for community engagement - the Five Elements model;
- how to develop voluntary organisations, community groups, charities and social enterprises as strategic partners;
- establishing a 'list of lists' register to systematically reduce the risk of Seasonal Excess Deaths in vulnerable older people;
- how to develop tobacco control plans to have optimal impact on health inequalities in the shorter term.

---

[1]   http://www.hinstassociates.co.uk/page/useful-resources

Workbooks

The 'Christmas tree' diagnostic tool was used in a series of workshops to explore what blockages there were to people in most need accessing the health care services they required. A series of workbooks was produced to stimulate local partners to question whether the different aspects of demand for services and their supply were giving the optimal impact to the most disadvantaged populations. The workbooks were developed as an iterative learning tool through these local workshops, building on effective practice that emerged. A full set is available on the NHS Institute for Innovation and Improvement website.[2] They cover the following topics:

- generic workbook;
- cancer;
- stroke *(coming soon: awaiting gateway approval)*;
- diabetes;
- chronic obstructive pulmonary disease (COPD);
- infant mortality;
- tobacco control;
- alcohol harm reduction;
- employment, worklessness and health;
- offender health.

A number of these, such as the cancer[3] workbook, have formed the basis of further guides through work with the national lead organisation.

[2] www.institute.nhs.uk/commissioning/general/health_inequalities_national_support_team_resources.html

[3] Cancer collaborative recommendations with National Cancer Action Team: http://ncat.nhs.uk/sites/default/files/HINST%20NCAT%20How%20to%20Cancer%20final%20_%2009032011.pdf

APPENDIX B

Conditions and descriptors for the QCA study

Table B.1: Cancers

Condition	Descriptor	Data source
Commissioning	Present: 'basic practice' (see Appendix C for further details) Absent: areas meeting better than basic practice criteria (see Appendix C for further details)	Questionnaire
Strategic partnership working	Present: basic or basic/good practice (see Appendix C for further details) Absent: good or exemplary practice (see Appendix C for further details)	Questionnaire
Public health workforce planning	Present: basic or basic/good practice (see Appendix C for further details) Absent: good or exemplary practice (see Appendix C for further details)	Questionnaire
Health Partnership reviews of progress	Present: reviews every six months, annually or not yet done Absent: monthly or quarterly reviews	Questionnaire
General working culture	Present: individual commitment and champions Absent: either a widely shared 'team player' spirit or good plans and systems	Questionnaire
Organisational Culture	Present: very or quite aspirational Absent: comfortable or complacent	Questionnaire
Index of Multiple Deprivation (IMD) score	Present: an IMD score of less than 31.15 Absent: an IMD score of 31.15 or higher	Office for National Statistics, IMD 2007 average score
Spend per head on cancer	Present: £86 per head or higher Absent: less than £86 per head	Department of Health statistics for 2005/06
Crime rate	Present: fewer than 64.5 offences per 1,000 population[2] Absent: 64.5 offences or higher per 1,000 population	
PCT rating 2004/05	Present: 3 star rating Absent: 1 and 2 star ratings	

[1]   Calculations based on raw populations and net expenditure for 2005/06

[2]   2005/06 data

Table B.2: CVD

Condition	Descriptor	Data source
Smoking cessation services	Present: areas meeting basic/good practice and above – provision has been mapped across the area and is available in a wide range of settings; prevalence data is collected and used to target services; and there is effective targeting of 'seldom seen, seldom heard' groups. Absent: basic practice – there is a multi-agency tobacco control alliance meeting regularly. GPs and nurses routinely advise smokers to quit and offer cessation support in at least 50% of practices/community pharmacies.	Questionnaire
Primary care services	Present: areas meeting basic/good practice and above – the PCT actively manages QOF exception reporting; primary care works with other services to reach vulnerable groups and to actively seek out people with (or at risk of) diseases; and the quantity of primary care in local areas meets local needs. Absent: basic practice – achievements against standards are audited and satisfactory. There are mechanisms for identifying poor performance and recovery plans.	Questionnaire
Approaches to tackling the CVD gap	Present: a few major programmes Absent: many smaller projects or integrated systematic approach	Questionnaire
Leadership in the Spearhead area	Present: good or excellent Absent: fair, poor or a mixed picture	Questionnaire
PCT target budget allocation	Present: PCTs receiving no less than 4.3% under their 2005/06 target budget Absent: PCTs receiving more than 4.3% under their 2005/06 PCT target budget	Department of Health statistics for 2005/06
Internal migration[3]	Present: lower levels of internal migration Absent: higher levels of internal migration	Statistics.gov.uk

[3]   This condition is derived from estimates of internal migration within the UK. The estimates are based on levels of both population inflow and outflow for each local authority in 2005/06. When dichotomised, the local authorities falling within the higher and lower inflow migration thresholds were exactly the same as those within the higher and lower outflow migration thresholds. Therefore, a single 'internal migration' condition is used. The migration threshold corresponds to 3.6% for population inflow and 4% for population outflow.

Table B.3: Teenage conceptions

Condition	Descriptor	Data source
Good or exemplary commissioning of local services	Present: 'basic practice', with plans and contracts in place and addressing differential needs, who manages what identified, and local managers meeting regularly. There is consultation across all stakeholders about improving services, especially among at risk groups. Absent: areas meeting basic practice criteria but with, in addition, joint plans, budgets and planning across services, with services commissioned on the basis of a sexual health needs assessment, and resources directed at 'hotspots' and prevention.	Questionnaire
Interventions all or mostly in community settings	Present: interventions focus on community settings where young people live and spend their spend leisure time. Absent: interventions focus on school and college settings.	Questionnaire
Fair or poor leadership	Present: leadership of tackling teenage pregnancies in the area is fair, poor or a mixed picture. Absent: leadership is good or excellent.	Questionnaire
Focus on a few major programmes	Present: the area's approach is based on a few major programmes to reduce teenage pregnancy rates. Absent: The area's approach is based on many smaller projects or a mixed approach.	Questionnaire
Lower numbers in drug treatment	Present: Number of individuals recorded as in drug treatment is less than 570 per 100,000. Absent: Number of individuals in treatment is 570 per 100,000 or higher.	Department of Health statistics for 2005/06
Higher educational achievement (GCSE subject passes)	Present: more than 96.65% of students in the area achieved at least one GCSE subject pass. Absent: 96.65% or fewer students achieved at least one GCSE pass.	Department for Education and Skills statistics for 2005/06
Higher percentage of under-18s	Present: more than 24% of the area's population is under 18. Absent: 24% or less of the population is under 18.	2001 census
Higher minority ethnic population	Present: the local authority area's minority ethnic population equals or exceeds 12.8% as a proportion of the total population. Absent: the local authority area's minority ethnic population is less than 12.8% as a proportion of the total population.	2001 census
Lower deprivation	Present: the IMD score for the area is less than 30.9. Absent: the IMD score is 30.9 or higher.	Office for National Statistics, IMD 2007 average score

Bureaucratic conditions for cancers QCA results

Table C.1: Bureaucratic conditions for cancers QCA results

	Public health workforce	Partnership working at strategic level	The role of commissioning	Frequency of progress reviews
Less than basic				Not yet done
Basic	A well-skilled, staffed and resourced public health workforce is in place to tackle the cancers gap.	A local strategic partnership with appropriate representation that receives progress reports from a health partnership/sub-group is established; a cancer network is established.	Existing plans and contracts address inequalities. Who manages what is identified, services accommodate referral-to-treatment targets and the impact on capacity is accommodated.	Annually
Good	As 'basic', plus includes clear link between local plans and capacity and skill levels. There is clear leadership of workforce planning. New types of worker are introduced to reach high risk groups.	As 'basic', plus there is strong leadership of the agenda and mainstreaming through a local area agreement, and an evidence-based health strategy with an action plan, targets, timelines, identified roles and data sharing. Plans are aligned and delivery coordinated across agencies.	All of 'basic', plus services are commissioned and networked, with cancer inequalities prioritised. Delays in patient pathways are addressed. Contracts are aligned and there is some budget pooling and joint contracting. There are lead project managers for specific tasks. User involvement, community campaigns and staff training are resourced to support appropriate use of services.	Quarterly

	Public health workforce	Partnership working at strategic level	The role of commissioning	Frequency of progress reviews
Exemplary	As 'good', plus there is effective pooled capacity across agencies, workforce plans embrace all sectors and long-term plans develop the right skills mix and capacity. Implementation is performance managed. There is a shared intelligence function for service planning and performance monitoring.	As 'good', plus there are shared/pooled resources and joint planning and contracting. Partners account for progress. Health inequality impact assessment is used. The cancer network has developed all aspects of cancer services.	All of 'good', plus resources are clearly scaled up to narrow the cancer gap based on targets, modelling and commissioning at scale. There are joint plans, processes, contracts, and management and information systems across all stakeholders. Service standards are explicitly detailed in service level agreements.	Monthly

Index

Note: Page numbers in *italic* type refer to tables or diagrams.